E Dr. Citron's volutionary Diet and Cookbook

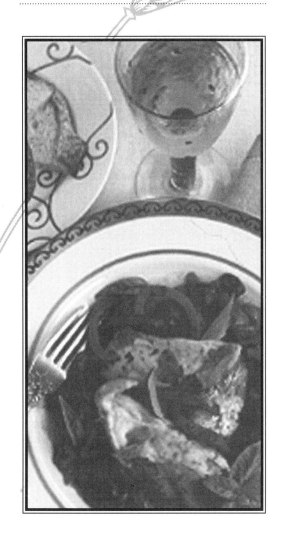

Advance Praise for Dr. Citron's
Evolutionary Diet and Cookbook

❈ ❈ ❈

"The information in this book will improve Quality of Life and the Health Status of the population."

— Michael Bendon, M.D., Vice President, Provider Support, Allina Health Care Systems

❈ ❈ ❈

"Dr. Citron's Evolutionary Diet and Cookbook is a delicious pill to swallow."

— David Fittingoff, M.D., Diplomate, American Board of Endocrinology

❈ ❈ ❈

"Great recipes for the amateur chef and the serious cook."

— Fred Halpert, Chef-Owner, Brava Terrace, St. Helena, CA James Beard Foundation, National Advisory Board

❈ ❈ ❈

"HEARTfelt congratulations on a life-saving book."

— Harvey Alpern, M.D., Fellow, American College of Cardiology

❈ ❈ ❈

"Microbiologically sound!"

— Dr. Maria Appleman, Director of Microbiology, USC Laboratories

❈ ❈ ❈

"A [R]Evolutionary book for your health."

— Peter N.R. Heseltine, M.D., Professor of Medicine, University of Southern California

Please visit the Hay House Website at:
http://www.hayhouse.com

Dr. Citron's Evolutionary Diet and Cookbook

Help Prevent Cancer and Heart Disease— and Lose Weight Naturally— by Following the Diet of Your Cro-Magnon Ancestors!

Ronald S. Citron, M.D.,
and
Kathye J. Citron

Hay House, Inc.
Carlsbad, CA

Published and distributed in the United States by:
Hay House, Inc., P.O. Box 5100, Carlsbad, CA 92018-5100 • (800) 654-5126 • (800) 650-5115 (fax)

Edited by: Jill Kramer   Designed by: Christy Allison
Cover Photo: Barry J. Blau Photography
Food Stylist: Kimberly Huson
Interior Food Photos: Peter J. Kaplan

The authors of this book do not dispense medical advice or prescribe the use of any technique as a form of treatment for physical or medical problems without the advice of your own physician, either directly or indirectly. The intent of the authors is only to offer information of a general nature to help you in your quest for emotional well-being and good health. In the event you use any of the information in this book for yourself, which is your constitutional right, the authors and the publisher assume no responsibility for your actions.

Library of Congress Cataloging-in-Publication Data

Citron, Ronald S.
    [Evolutionary diet and cookbook]
    Dr. Citron's evolutionary diet and cookbook : help prevent cancer and heart disease—and lose weight naturally—by following the diet of your Cro-Magnon ancestors! / Ronald S. Citron and Kathye J. Citron.
        p.   cm.
    Includes bibliographical references and index.
    ISBN 1-56170-354-0   FRom BAcK CoVER/ISBN 1 - 56170 - 522 - 5 (pbK)
    1. Diet in disease.   2. Man, Primitive—Food.   3. Human evolution.   4. Cancer—Prevention.
5. Coronary heart disease—Prevention.   6. Reducing diets—Recipes.   I. Title.
    RM216.C5764   1997
    613.2—dc20
                                                                                    96-33164
                                                                                    CIP

ISBN 1-56170-354-0

00 99 98 97   4 3 2 1
First Printing, March 1997

Printed in the United States of America

To

Louis Camille Maillard and Alice Waters:
Persons of Good Taste

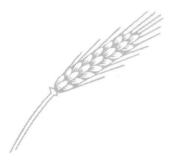

Authors' Note

Dr. Citron's Evolutionary Diet and Cookbook is not meant to act as a substitute for professional health care. Any decision that you make involving your health, or the treatment of an illness, should include the specific advice of your personal medical doctor. The information in this book is general. We hope you will use it for your good health and to increase your knowledge. Yet, since all of us are unique, we hope that the knowledge you gain will enable you to interface with your health-care professionals in an even more efficient and informed manner on specific health issues. Please do not change your diet if you are seriously ill without first discussing it with your doctor. Do not change medications without professional advice.

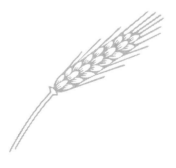

Contents

PART III: APPENDIX

❖ ❖ ❖ ❖ ❖ ❖

Acknowledgments

S ome people may think that it's easy to write a book. We found that more work goes into the final product than we had ever imagined. During the writing of this book, and the tasting and testing of the recipes, we enlisted the help of a great many people. They are individuals who gave of their time and expertise freely, with love, genuine concern, and caring for this project. If we named everyone, we would have an acknowledgment section as long as a chapter. So, we thank all of you who touched this work, and mention below only a few special people who spent considerable time and energy on the book.

We thank: Louise Hay, who had the prescience to realize that medical self-help has become an extremely important part of health care; Reid Tracy, who "makes it all happen"; Jill Kramer, our editor, catlover, and believer in miracles, who picked our manuscript out of the piles on her desk, saw potential in it, and put it into final form; Christy Allison, designer and risk taker; and the entire staff at Hay House, a truly remarkable group of dedicated, gracious, kind, and warm people.

We thank Barry "Barton" Blau, who had the dignity to endure constant dinners at 10 P.M. or later, where he tasted all of these fabulous (and some not-so-fabulous) dishes before they were in final form. He tirelessly and generously came to our rescue in many guises: as our cover photographer, photo editor, food tester, and friend.

We thank our family and friends who spent countless hours reading and rereading the text and testing the recipes. Many of their suggestions have been incorporated into the book. We especially wish to thank: Donna Beltz; Gary Block; Bud and Gloria Bradley; Steve Gelman; Peter N.R. Heseltine, M.D.; Deborah Mason; Richard McCarty; Paul Miller; Karen Murphy; Dr. Peter Nagourney; Don Sefton; Trip Sternburgh; Van Sternburgh; and Ben and Sherry Tunnell.

We thank Peter J. Kaplan, long-time friend and food photographer who traveled from New York to Los Angeles to "shoot" our food.

We thank Paul Mercado and Marlene Ricigliano of Crate & Barrel for their efficiency and graciousness while helping us put together settings for the food shots.

And last, but far from least, we thank our serendipitous angel, Wendy Dale (soon-to-be famous scriptwriter), who helped change some medical mutterings into readable prose; and John Gibson Miller (soon-to-be famous actor), our food tester and taster.

PART I
What Is the Evolutionary Diet?

Introduction

This Book May Save Your Life

Imagine this: A doctor tells you that you can lose weight and live to be active and in good shape until you're 100 years old (at least). All you have to do is eat a diet of mashed yeast, bean sprouts, and sunflower seeds for the rest of your life. Could you do it? Personally, I couldn't. Three days on that diet and I'd be willing to give up years of my life for just one serving of lobster, a plate of pasta, or a piece of pie.

That's the problem with most diet plans. They're simply impossible to stick with. How many people do you know who are still on the Rotation Diet, the Immune Power Diet, or the Beverly Hills Diet?

As a medical doctor, I've seen many of my patients try to change their eating habits after their first heart attack or the discovery that they have cancer. Scared, and willing to try almost anything that the medical world has to offer, they embark on a low-fat diet plan. But adhering to a very limited and unpalatable regimen is simply impossible. And eventually, the "beef-attacks" set in, and these people cheat or go off the diet completely.

The truth is, the more restrictive a diet is, the sooner you will give it up. But luckily, you don't have to choose between enjoying delicious foods and maintaining good health. In this book, you'll find guidelines for healthy eating—for people who love to eat. You're not going to have to make radical lifestyle changes, and you're not going to have to deprive yourself. In fact, your food preferences may become even more exotic.

Most important, by eating a diet that's in sync with your genes, you'll decrease your risk of getting cancer and heart disease. You'll gain health and vitality and prolong your life. As an added benefit, by feeding your body the foods it needs, you'll also lose weight.

This book will do more than change your life—it may just *save* it.

How This Book Came to Be

As a medical oncologist—a cancer specialist—I spent years battling one of the toughest diseases known to human beings. Patient after patient came into my office dying of an illness that was, in part, caused by poor eating habits.

I realized that I could do more good *preventing* this disease, rather than just trying to help patients once it was too late. So, I began researching and cataloging the effects that certain risk factors, including foods, had on a person's health, and I noticed an interesting connection: The foods that helped prevent cancer were the same as those that could protect against heart disease. Similarly, the foods most blamed for contributing to heart disease were those most often associated with cancer.

This finding raised some interesting questions. Why could some foods prevent illness while others were so life-threatening? Why did the human body not only refuse to metabolize certain foods properly, but actually behave as if it were being poisoned?

After much research and thought, I began to understand the answers to these questions. We, as a species, had outwitted evolution. We, unlike any other animals, had developed the ability to change our environment. Along with inventing automobiles, ketchup, light bulbs, and underwear, we had begun creating new types of foods—processed foods full of fat that Nature never intended us to eat. And this was killing us—because we had not yet evolved the genes to metabolize these foods. Our cultural evolution had moved faster than our genetic evolution.

Having finally grasped the problem, one night while preparing a meal,

I was struck by the solution. *I realized that we should be eating the same foods that our early Cro-Magnon ancestors ate.* Comparing their lifestyle and diet to more contemporary hunter-gatherers convinced me that it was unlikely that they suffered from heart disease and cancer, yet they ate lots of red meat, nuts, eggs, and shellfish and other high-cholesterol foods that we frown upon today.

At first, the thought merely amused me: Go back to nuts and berries, and start a nomadic life living off the land. It was the kind of idea that novels or cults or fad diets are made of—it was hardly a serious thought. But as I pondered the problem further, I realized that we really could replicate the diet of the Cro-Magnons, our Stone Age ancestors.

Using my medical knowledge and experience as a physician, I began by creating what I knew to be an anti-cancer, anti-heart disease diet. Then I began to do research. Books on ethnology and anthropology validated my thinking: The diet of our ancient ancestors truly was the ideal anti-cancer, anti-heart disease diet!

I continued by studying the diets of primitive hunter-gatherer tribes still in existence today. These people are eating like our ancestors and, interestingly enough, they are incredibly healthy, with no heart disease or cancer.

Then, I set about creating a menu. Luckily, I live in Los Angeles, a city of great ethnic diversity, so I began exploring every market I could, studying the cuisine and finding the ingredients that comprised the foods of Japan, China, India, Korea, France, Greece, and other countries.

That knowledge, combined with my wife's and my own professional cooking experience and our love of food, enabled us to transform ordinary foods, usually prepared without imagination or flavor, into attractive, savory dishes that are as healthful as they are delicious.

That's how this book first came to be. Naming the diet was the final step. I decided to call it the Evolutionary Diet because, by following it, you will undergo a personal evolution in your eating habits, and you'll properly feed your 30,000-year-old genes.

What the Evolutionary Diet Can Do for You

So what exactly am I promising you? We'll start with weight loss, since it's the least important benefit of the Evolutionary Diet, yet the easiest to achieve.

Without counting calories or portions, your weight will drop—simply because you are giving your body the foods it needs, the foods it is best suited to metabolize.

When I first met Kathye, the woman who would later become my wife, we spent much of our time together preparing and eating new creations. (She is a chef who owned a catering business, and I have worked in professional kitchens.) Together, we'd make meals based on the Evolutionary Diet principles, and after three months, Kathye told me that she'd never felt better. Without counting calories or trying to lose weight, she had dropped seven pounds.

If weight loss is your goal, the Evolutionary Diet will help you achieve it—but there is a much more important benefit. Follow the guidelines outlined in this book, and you'll feel healthier and be able to live well into old age. If you avoid illness, your organ systems can function for well over a century—which means that you could live to be more than 100 years old.

Eating properly will decrease your risk of getting some of the most common cancers (including colon, prostate, bladder, esophagus, stomach, and pancreas) by at least 80 percent. It will also decrease your risk of heart and arterial disease, hypertension, and stroke by a great degree.

What's a Cro-Magnon to Eat?

The Evolutionary Diet isn't just about nuts and berries. Let me give you some idea of what you'll be eating:

How about gazpacho for a light lunch or salmon with Japanese spices, a seasonal green salad, and sorbet with dried fruit compote for dessert? Try some tomatillo soup, and follow it with delicious seafood-smoked shrimp, or sample grilled marinated squab with sage potatoes plus a salad of fennel and endives. Enjoy swordfish with Mexican salsa, or serve coriander chicken with a side of California ratatouille.

Not hungry yet? Then try roasted rabbit with pineapple/mustard sauce, grilled snapper with ginger "butter," or venison carpaccio.

Desserts are no less intriguing: figs in cognac, fruit terrine, and banana puree with dates and nuts.

If I've succeeded in whetting your appetite, go ahead and peek at the recipes in the second half of the book. Or jump right in and try one.

30,000-Year-Old Food:
Better Than a Fresh Hamburger

Why is a diet that's 30,000 years old actually better for us than what we're eating today? The answer is simple: Our genes haven't changed in 30,000 years, but our eating habits have. What that means is that we're trying to digest fast-food hamburgers and fries using a Cro-Magnon metabolism. And eating that way is killing us. Our industrialized urban culture has brought with it a diet made up of foods that are processed, high in dairy products, loaded with fat, and full of salt. As a result, we suffer from two crippling and fatal ailments—cancer and heart disease—which were never in nature's game plan.

But if we look at individuals in primitive societies who attained the age of 55, we see something quite different. They had a firm foundation of good health. There was no hardening of the arteries, no cancer. One of the main differences between them and us is...diet.

So how do we know what the Stone Age diet was like? How do we know that this diet was the secret of the hunter-gatherers' good health? Although prehistoric people left no written record to tell us anything about their health, they did leave us their remains. By measuring strontium levels in hunter-gatherers' bones and examining artifacts and animal bones that were found at dwelling sites, scientists began to develop a clear picture of how Cro-Magnons ate and lived.

These ancient people were primarily hunter-gatherers (agriculture hadn't been discovered back then), so they subsisted on what they found and what they killed. They gathered nuts, fruits, berries, and vegetables, and found seeds and grains in small amounts. The rest of their diet was made up of wild animal meat. They caught birds, rodents, and other mammals, and probably ate some eggs. Tribes living by rivers or seas also had fish and shellfish.

It was a diet high in protein, high in carbohydrates, and most important for us, very low in fat.

Wait a minute, you say. All that meat—is that really healthy? How could the Cro-Magnon diet possibly be low in fat?

It's true that most meat you'll find in the grocery store today is very high in fat. But our Cro-Magnon ancestors weren't shopping in supermarkets; they were eating animals that they had hunted. And this wild game was low in overall fat content as well as saturated fat.

Today, we breed our livestock to be very high in fat (supposedly because it makes the meat more tender). A steer raised on a farm is at least 25 percent fat by weight. But a deer living in the wild is only four percent fat by weight. That means that two pounds of wild venison have less fat than half a pound of steak.

At this point, you may be concerned that I'm going to tell you that you're going to have to go and kill your own dinner or that you'll have to eat nothing but wild deer meat for the rest of your life. Don't worry. There are plenty of other sources of meat available (such as crustaceans, bivalves, fish, chicken, and commercially available wild game) that are good for you and low in fat.

In chapter four, I'll tell you more about these healthful sources of protein.

How Do We Know It Was Diet That Kept Our Cro-Magnon Ancestors So Healthy?

Modern hunter-gatherer tribes who eat much like their Cro-Magnon ancestors (such as the ¡Kung-San, and the Kade of Africa) were studied in the '60s and found to be in remarkably good health. Their blood cholesterol levels averaged 120 milligrams, about half the average cholesterol level in the U.S. Their blood pressure was low and remained low (unlike most Americans—whose blood pressure gradually rises with age). Scientists found no heart disease, no coronary artery disease, no angina, and no incidence of heart attacks (and subjects up to 83 years of age were examined). There were also no cases of diabetes.

Unfortunately, since these initial studies were conducted 30 years ago, the ¡Kung-San and other tribes have become influenced by Western lifestyles. They have increased their intake of saturated fat. And as their diets have changed, their health has deteriorated.

A very similar pattern has also emerged among the Australian aborigines. In the wild, aborigines (who eat a diet very closely resembling the Evolutionary Diet) have a very low incidence of diabetes, cardiovascular disease, and cancer. However, those who have integrated into the white

Australian population (and have begun consuming a high-fat, high saturated-fat diet) have developed appreciable rates of these diseases.

Eating a high-fat diet goes hand in hand with increasing one's risk for hardening of the arteries and cancer. Nowhere today is this relationship more striking than in the Japanese. Several decades ago, Japanese women living in Japan had very low rates of breast cancer. But Japanese women who moved to Hawaii (and started eating more like Americans) developed a higher incidence of the disease, and Japanese women who lived in Los Angeles were at a still greater risk. Why? Scientists explain that this phenomenon resulted largely from dietary changes.

Also in Japan, rates of cancer of the large intestine have increased. As the Japanese have become more affluent and have adopted Western eating preferences (steak, for example), the incidence of colon cancer and breast cancer has risen to an alarming degree. Rates of heart disease and hardening of the arteries have also become major health problems.

What can we learn from these observations? *A high-fat, high saturated-fat diet is associated with an increased risk for cancer and heart disease. On the other hand, a low-fat diet of mostly unsaturated fat (the Evolutionary Diet) is one of the keys to avoiding these diseases.*

I'll go into more detail in upcoming chapters.

Evidence from Closer to Home

Instead of evaluating primitive hunter-gatherers, let's examine some groups of people living in the United States whose diet resembles the Evolutionary Diet.

The Mormons, who do not smoke or drink and eat a diet low in domesticated, or commercially raised red meat, have a strikingly low incidence of cancer. Not only do they show reduced rates of the types of cancer associated with alcohol and tobacco use (such as cancer of the lungs, mouth, throat, larynx, pancreas, kidney, and esophagus), they also have a lower incidence of cancers of the breast, large intestine, and prostate. And, they have a markedly lower incidence of cancer of the cervix and the central nervous system.

Seventh Day Adventists have a longer life expectancy and lower morbidity (rate of sickness) than the general population. Why? Because their religion advocates a diet free from alcohol, tobacco, and meat. Studies conducted between practicing and nonpracticing Seventh Day Adventists show a very strong correlation between meat consumption and hardening of the arteries. Meat eaters had rates of heart disease 300 percent higher than non-meat eaters!

As you would probably expect, Seventh Day Adventists who stick to a diet free from meat, alcohol, and tobacco also show appreciably lower incidences of cancer. (Isn't it interesting how the risks for cancer and heart disease always go together?) The incidence of cancer of the lower intestine and the prostate are especially low for these practicing Adventists.

Similarly, vegetarians, who eat a diet very low in total fat (most of which is unsaturated), have little hardening of the arteries, low death rates from heart attack, and a low incidence of common cancers.

All of this evidence points to a simple fact:

THE FIRST AND MOST IMPORTANT STEP TO AVOIDING CANCER AND HEART DISEASE IS TO REDUCE THE AMOUNT OF FAT (ESPECIALLY SATURATED FAT) IN YOUR DIET.

I thought that I was really on to something very important: a unified theory of sickness based on the difference between the slow pace of biologic evolution and our fast-forwarded civilization.

BUT THERE WAS MORE! By the time I had finished my research, I had also learned additional information regarding:

❋ The relationship between cholesterol measured in our diet and cholesterol measured in our blood. It turns out that these two are not related to one another at all. In fact, eating high-cholesterol foods can actually *lower* blood cholesterol! Astounding as this may seem, there is a reason for this, which I will explain in chapter two.

❋ The "problem" with protein. Most health and diet books advise a lower protein intake than is required by our bodies. My research indicates that we are naturally inclined to eat the right amount of protein, more than is advised by many health and nutrition "gurus."

 <u>Several very important findings in the field of childhood nutrition</u>. From the viewpoint of the Evolutionary Diet, how and what we eat as infants and children is critically important in determining our future health. Even many young children already have the early signs of **hardening of the arteries!** We will have more to say about this important area in chapter seven. But first, we'd better start at the beginning....

Chapter One
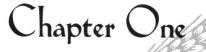

Evolution and
Why We Get Sick

In 30,000 years, a lot has changed. While our Cro-Magnon ancestors concerned themselves with hunting mastodon, creating a few cave drawings, and hoping someone would hurry up and invent the wheel, we live in an era of technology, transportation, and communication—a time of cars and planes and computers—of fast food and Ziploc bags and cappuccino-flavored frozen yogurt.

As much as our culture has changed throughout time, our bodies have remained pretty much the same. We have essentially the same genetic makeup as our ancestors of 30,000 years ago—which means that our metabolism works in basically the same way.

The problem is, we have bodies that are ideally suited to digest mastodon, berries, and seeds—but we're consuming greasy hamburgers, fries, and chocolate shakes. And eating that way is creating a host of health problems.

To understand why this is so, you have to know something about the way evolution works.

A Cliff Notes *Guide to Evolution*

Evolution, simply stated, is the adaptation of a species to its environment. It's the reason why bears living in the cold have furry coats (to keep them warm), why plants living in the desert have thick waxy skins (to keep from drying out), and why horses grazing in the fields are able to digest hay and grass (pretty handy when you're already walking around in the stuff all day).

Evolution, stated another way, is the force that "puts us in sync" with our surroundings. But if we're in sync, why aren't we able to safely eat fast and processed foods—foods that are so omnipresent in our environment?

The simple answer is that genetic evolution is very slow, a process that takes much longer than cultural change. Let me explain.

When the theory of evolution was first being put forth, it was incorrectly assumed that an *individual* could adapt to its environment. That is to say, put a hairless polar bear into the snow, and magically it would adapt by suddenly growing fur.

But evolution doesn't work that way. It can't change an *individual;* it can only change a *species.* It works according to what Darwin termed "survival of the fittest."

A polar bear won't magically grow fur if it's put out in the cold, but if you put 100 polar bears in the snow, the ones that have the warmest coats will be the ones to survive. And the survivors, the "fittest members of the species," will pass on the fur-coat trait to their offspring. So after a while ("a while" in evolutionary time being hundreds of thousands of years), nearly all polar bears will have thick, warm coats.

Environmental conditions are constantly changing—in this example, a warm area is growing colder. And when these natural changes occur, evolution kicks in, eliminating the weakest individuals and causing a species to adapt to its changing environment.

What Do Fuzzy Bears Have to Do with My Health?

Being in sync with your environment doesn't just mean keeping warm. It also means being able to eat the foods your environment provides.

Evolution is the reason why koalas eat eucalyptus (since they live in the trees) and dolphins (since they live in the ocean) eat fish. Evolution is the reason why we as humans can eat fruits, vegetables, grains, and meat. But dairy products and fast and processed foods are also part of our lives. Why haven't we evolved to be able to eat these foods and stay healthy?

The simplest explanation is that evolution hasn't had the time to catch up with our current environment. In evolutionary terms, the appearance of these "bad foods" is very recent.

To give you some idea of the time it takes for evolution to create a change in DNA, let's compress the history of the entire universe into one year. In other words, we'll say that the universe was created at midnight on January 1st. On this time scale, the human race wouldn't even have appeared until December 31 of that year at 10:30 P.M. The Bronze Age would have started the same day at 11:59:56 P.M. (that's four seconds before midnight), and the Renaissance would have started on the same day at 11:59:59 P.M. (that's one second before midnight). Keep in mind that DNA changes take hundreds of thousands to millions of years to occur. At this rate, a significant evolutionary change wouldn't appear until around 1:00 A.M. on January 1 of the next year (that is, an hour later).

Looking at time in this way makes us realize how young we humans are in the scheme of the universe. Yet at the same time, we have been incredibly successful in populating the Earth. Over the past 2,000 years, our numbers have increased dramatically. See Figure 1A, which charts world population since A.D. zero. The explosive growth of our numbers puts added stresses on our ability to gather and distribute food. The more of us there are, the more difficult it becomes to eat "naturally."

Figure 1A

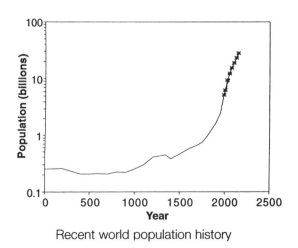

Recent world population history

If we can't solve our population problem, and assuming we had all the time in the world, will we eventually evolve and develop the genes to process saturated fat?

At first thought, it seems that the answer would be yes. Anyone who has this gene has a much better chance of surviving, so in theory, given millions of years, this advantage should be passed on.

However, evolution makes changes in a species through reproduction. (In other words, the fittest members of a species reproduce, and the least fit members die before they can pass on their weak genetic makeups to their offspring.) But in our case, this genetic flaw doesn't manifest itself until *after* we have children. Heart attacks and cancer occur later in life, giving us plenty of time to pass on this defect.

What's DNA Got to Do with It?

DNA (deoxyribonucleic acid) is our genetic material. We have the same genetic makeup as our Cro-Magnon ancestors because their DNA has been passed on to us (children inherit their DNA from their parents) over 30,000 years.

It's important to understand how DNA works because it determines everything that we are physically (or can become)—it is the blueprint for our bodies. Within DNA lies the code not only for the color of our eyes, the shape of our noses, and the thickness of our hair, but DNA also controls the way our bodies process food.

DNA acts very much like a computer program. Just as a word processor can't perform math calculations, your DNA can't do anything for which it was not programmed. If the genes are not present to do a particular job, it can't be done. As a result of evolution, most of us do not have the genes to process saturated fat, but because of our culture, saturated fat is practically being crammed into us. And that's the reason we're dying from heart disease, heart attacks, and many forms of cancer.

You've probably heard the expression "Garbage In, Garbage Out." This is true not only for computer programs, but for humans as well. If we eat garbage (that is, foods that our bodies are not genetically adapted to metabolize), our bodies will not function properly. But if we consume the right stuff (the foods our bodies are programmed to digest), our bodies will perform at their optimal best.

So, we're stuck with the genetic makeup of a Cro-Magnon. The good news is, if you know how your metabolism works, you can feed your body the foods it's best suited to digest. And if you feed your body the foods it needs, you'll not only be able to enjoy the life you have, you'll have a lot longer life to enjoy (not to mention the fact that you'll also lose weight).

Taking care of your body is very similar to taking care of the tires on your car. Drive normally, and your tires will wear normally. But if you continually hit potholes when you drive, or if you fail to get your car aligned, the life of your tires will be shortened and they won't work well most of the time.

Just as a car's tires show tread wear, our parts eventually wear out, too. This can't be changed; wear and tear are part of the order of things. But disease is not a natural part of growing old. Remember, if you avoid disease, your organs can keep functioning for 100 years or more.

You can't live forever, but you can live longer, and you can achieve your ideal weight. You can be healthier, happier, and more fulfilled if you pay attention to what your body needs. The key is to eat foods that you can most easily digest and metabolize. And it's very important that you begin establishing healthy eating habits *now*.

The point to remember is this:

WE HAVE THE SAME GENES AS OUR
30,000-YEAR-OLD ANCESTORS.
ALTHOUGH WE CAN'T CHANGE OUR GENES,
WE *CAN* CHANGE OUR DIET.

Chapter Two

Dietary Cholesterol Doesn't Count

W hen I first began my research into the diets of our early Cro-Magnon ancestors, I came upon an interesting mystery: Hunter-gatherers living today (in Borneo, Africa, New Guinea, and other countries) were eating the same amount of cholesterol found in our Western diet, yet their blood cholesterol was half the level of most Americans! This meant that although they were eating just as much cholesterol-filled food as we were, it wasn't hurting them in the same way that it was hurting us. Being a doctor, naturally I was very interested in how this could be.

After much research and thought, I finally came upon the solution to this mystery: It wasn't the amount of cholesterol in the diet that mattered; it was the *saturated fat* we were eating. Simply defined, saturated fat is any fat that hardens at room temperature. Think of bacon grease, and you've got the picture. Saturated fats are found in abundance in animal products. Domesticated meats (especially red meat) and all dairy products that are not nonfat (including cheese, milk, yogurt, and butter) are all high in saturated fat.

Unsaturated fat is found in plant foods, poultry, fish, and wild game.

This is the "good fat"—not that you can just eat chicken and drink olive oil all day. The point is, unsaturated fats are not bad for you when consumed in reasonable quantities.

What Is Cholesterol Anyway?

Contrary to popular belief, cholesterol is not a fat. Cholesterol is a molecule that's found in every cell in your body. In fact, any amount of cholesterol that you could eat is a very small fraction of the total amount that already exists in your body. Cholesterol is essential to the proper functioning of your organs. It's necessary because it helps make up the cell membrane, the "skin" that holds everything in the cell together.

Just as cholesterol is found in your body, it makes up the cell membrane in other animals as well. Of course, this includes the animals we eat. Eat lobster or steak or fish, and you're consuming cholesterol.

A great misperception in nutritional counseling is the confusion between the amount of cholesterol in the diet and the amount of cholesterol in the blood. They are two totally different issues. For years, doctors have been admonishing their patients not to eat *any* foods containing cholesterol. But just how bad are these foods? In actuality, they're not bad at all if they do not contain saturated fat. There are many foods that are high in cholesterol and low in fat. They are: crustaceans (lobster, crab, shrimp, crayfish) and bivalves (clams, oysters, mussels). Keep in mind that while three ounces of lean hamburger and three ounces of lobster meat contain the same amount of cholesterol (about 85 mg.), a hamburger has almost *19 times more fat* (15 gm. vs. 0.8 gm.)! So, eating a high cholesterol (and low-in-saturated fat) lobster will have almost no effect on your blood cholesterol, but eating the same amount of high-cholesterol (and high-in-saturated fat) hamburger will have a greater impact on your blood cholesterol (and your weight). Why is this true?

Cholesterol *by itself* doesn't cause your body any problems. It's metabolized and goes to work performing essential functions. But cholesterol doesn't ever travel by itself. It's like the cargo in a boat—it has to be transported in your body attached to something else. And the type of "boat" blood cholesterol travels in is related to the type of fat you eat. If cholesterol is traveling in a "boat" that is created in response to eating unsaturated fat, there's no problem. Unsaturated fat doesn't cause your body any damage; in fact, it helps to unclog blocked arteries. But if the cholesterol is traveling in a "boat" created from eating saturated fat, your body is in for a vicious attack. Saturated fat releases cholesterol in the walls of the arteries (where you definitely don't want cholesterol to be!). On the other hand, unsaturated fat safely releases cholesterol into the liver, where it can be processed.

HIGH-CHOLESTEROL FOODS BY THEMSELVES DO
NOT RAISE YOUR CHOLESTEROL LEVEL. IN ORDER
FOR CHOLESTEROL TO BE HARMFUL, IT
MUST BE EATEN WITH SATURATED FAT.

So, you don't need to worry about how much cholesterol you're consuming; what you need to do is limit your intake of saturated fat. This means that you can eat all the (cholesterol-filled) lobster you want as long as you don't dip it in butter (which is high in saturated fat), because cholesterol *by itself* is not harmful.

When you eat cholesterol, one of several things can happen: If your body can metabolize it correctly, the cholesterol goes to work performing essential functions; what's left over is removed (mainly through the liver). But if you've eaten a diet high in saturated fat, it's very likely that the cholesterol will be deposited in your arteries and harden. This is called arteriosclerosis (hardening of the arteries), and it's to blame for a myriad of health problems.

It's easy to understand why arteriosclerosis is so dangerous. Imagine that your arteries are like the plumbing system in your house. Throw hair and grease down your drains, and eventually the water isn't going to make its way through the pipes. Your body works in much the same way. Clog up your arteries (by eating saturated fat), and your blood won't be able to circulate.

Understanding Arteriosclerosis

Arteriosclerosis (also called *atherosclerosis* or *hardening of the arteries*) begins with an injury to the inside lining of the arteries. This injury can be provoked by many things, the most common of which is stress caused by movement. Even bending your arm at your elbow causes the stretching and distorting of the blood vessels. Of course, this injury isn't serious and is quickly repaired by your body.

The injuries you need to worry about are the ones that are not easily fixed by your body. Luckily, these injuries can be prevented. They're caused by smoking, too much insulin (our bodies produce insulin when we eat sugar), high blood pressure, saturated fat, stress, and other factors (more on this subject in later chapters).

Once there's an injury to the inside lining of an artery, blood clots begin to form (in the same way as when you cut your finger). Clotting is necessary in order for your body to repair the damaged area; however, these blood clots are sticky so they easily attract other particles. (Notice how often hair and dirt get stuck in newly forming scabs.) Cholesterol, fat, and calcium adhere to the area, harden, and over time begin blocking vital arteries. As if this weren't bad enough, the problem begins to snowball. Once hardening of the arteries begins, cholesterol has a perfect platform to which it can adhere. So, hardening of the arteries promotes *further* hardening of the arteries.

Take a good look at a river, and you'll see similar forces at work. At curves in a river, sand gets built up on the inside of the bend and other areas of turbulent flow. Arteries follow the same basic rules. Injuries are most likely to form where there are bends and divisions of the vessels. Keep in mind that there are no straight arteries within your heart, and you will begin to see the extent of the danger. Arteriosclerosis is to blame for heart attacks, strokes, poor circulation, and a variety of other related health problems.

Those Lucky (and Not-So-Lucky) Genetic Mutants

"Wait a minute," you say. "All this talk about saturated fat. I have friends who eat nothing but saturated fat all day, and they're fine. How do you explain that?"

Well, I have a friend who does exactly the same thing. His name is Mark Kent and he's a doctor—a cardiologist, in fact! For breakfast, Mark eats two eggs, three to four slices of bacon, and potatoes cooked in grease. For lunch, it's often a hamburger and french fries, and his dinner is even worse! In the evening, he'll have pork dripping in grease, potatoes cooked in goose fat, and ice cream for dessert. Amazingly, Mark's cholesterol level is 160 (below 200 is considered healthy in an adult) *and* he is thin.

So what does Mark know that the rest of us don't? In this case, knowledge has nothing to do with it; Mark is simply exceptionally lucky. He has a genetic mutation that enables him to eat a diet high in saturated fat and successfully digest it.

Most of the rest of us don't have genes that can do the job of metabolizing these saturated fats. In fact, we'll never be able to accomplish this. Unlike lucky Mark and his genes, we aren't able to eat saturated fat without serious repercussions to our health.

But things could be worse. There is also a group of people who suffer from a disease called hyperlipoproteinemia. (Yes, that's really a word!) These people have a high cholesterol level even on a no-fat diet! They require medications to help get their blood cholesterol somewhere near the healthy range.

Fortunately, the rest of us can usually overcome the limitations of our genes through dietary management and by avoiding saturated fat.

You Can Begin Lowering Your Fat Intake Right Now

I was asked recently if there is any down side to avoiding saturated fat. At first I was surprised that anyone could ask this question, because the data relating saturated fats to illness is so strong. But on further reflection, I realized that it is a valid scientific concern. In fact, some physicians do argue that since the brain is composed of many different fatty acids, children should have a high fat intake for optimal brain development. However, *essential fatty acids*, needed for brain development, are present in fish oils and fatty fish. They are full of these vitally essential molecules—essential because they cannot be manufactured by the body (the nonessential fats are manufactured by us). We don't need to supplement a good evolutionary diet with high amounts of saturated fatty acids that are NOT essential. It's downright dangerous.

A group of scientists in Boston, for example, found that children who ate a predominantly vegetarian diet (whose diets were low in saturated fat) had IQs that were 20 percent above average. Other tests have shown that a high saturated-fat intake among children can be detrimental to their health. Children as young as ten have shown the early signs of hardening of the arteries. Other studies have shown that reducing the saturated fat intake even in young children lowers their serum cholesterol levels (more on this important point in chapter seven).

I am not advocating that you totally abstain from having fat in your diet. That would be impossible. Even lettuce has fat in it. But preventing fatal diseases such as arteriosclerosis and cancer means decreasing your overall consumption of fat—especially saturated fat.

In chapter nine, I'll show you how to watch your fat intake by learning to read nutritional labels. But don't wait until then to begin healthy eating. There are steps you can take right now to decrease the amount of fat you're consuming:

1. **Eliminate domesticated red meat from your diet.** All meat contains cholesterol, but not all meat is high in saturated fat. (Remember, it's saturated fat, not cholesterol, that we want to avoid.) Begin substituting wild red meat, game, poultry, crustaceans, and fish for domesticated red meat, and you're on your way to reducing the "bad fat" in your diet. We'll talk more about protein sources in chapter four.

2. **Eliminate all dairy foods that are not nonfat.** You've probably been told your whole life that milk is good for you, but except for the fact that it contains calcium, nothing could be further from the truth. High-fat dairy products are among our worst health enemies. Other than oils, they have more calories from fat than many other food sources, and they're filled with saturated fat. Nonfat dairy foods are the exceptions. These include nonfat: milk, yogurt, ricotta, and cottage cheese. (Unfortunately, there is no such thing as nonfat butter!) Try using these nonfat milk products in place of their unhealthy high-fat equivalents.

3. **Eliminate fast food.** Most fast food is loaded with excess fat. Not only that, it's usually processed so it has little nutritive value and gobs of salt. In place of that hamburger and fries, try making Asian Mushroom Soup, Smoked Chicken Risotto, or other dishes listed as "QUICK AND EASY" in the recipe section of this book.

If you are occasionally forced to eat at fast-food restaurants, look for those that now offer green salads with nonfat dressing or lemon juice; baked potatoes with salsa, barbeque sauce, or even catsup in place of butter or sour cream; and skinless, broiled (not breaded) chicken breast sandwiches. In desperation, I once ordered a hamburger and said, "Hold the mayo and the meat!"

4. **Eliminate "bad oils" from your diet.** No oils contain cholesterol (remember, cholesterol is found only in animal products), but there are several oils that are high in saturated fat. Try to eliminate these "bad oils" from your diet completely:

- all shortenings (even vegetable shortening is high in saturated fat)
- coconut oil
- palm oil
- palm kernel oil
- margarine

You may think it's no problem to avoid these high-saturated-fat foods because you don't cook with them; unfortunately, these "bad oils" are found in a multitude of packaged products including many candy bars, chocolates, cookies, and cakes. Anything hydrogenated or partially hydrogenated should be avoided. Read the labels!

In place of butter, shortening, and other oils high in saturated fat, try using these oils:

olive	peanut
mustard	corn
sesame	vegetable
sunflower	canola

However, a word of caution: Just because these "good oils" are low in saturated fat doesn't give you carte blanche in using them; the total amount of fat, even unsaturated fat, in your diet is very important. Oils contain more than twice the calories per gram than protein or carbohydrates (more on this later), so use oils very sparingly. Try thickening sauces with nonfat yogurt, cornstarch, mashed potato, pureed cooked rice, or even flour, and remember that truly flavorful oils can provide taste even when used in very small quantities. (See the recipes in section two of this book for examples.)

There Were No Obese Hunter-Gatherers

At this point, for your reading enjoyment, I offer the following short play to illustrate the way in which Cro-Magnons perceived their food:

From stage right, enter our hero Herb, an average Cro-Magnon male. He sits down on his favorite rock hoping to get a few minutes of much-needed rest. At stage left is Doris, his wife.

Doris: Herb, I'm starving. Go out and get us something to eat.

Herb: I thought that you still had that haunch of what I caught ten days ago.

Doris: But it's summer, and we haven't invented refrigeration yet. The meat was smelling, so I set it out for the pterodactyls. You know pterodactyls—they'll eat anything.

Herb: Yeah, those omnivores. What an appetite!

Doris: Plus the roots and seeds are almost gone. The kids are hungry, and so am I.

Herb: Okay Doris, I'll go out and try to find something, but my back still hurts from that mastodon escapade last winter so I probably won't get anything that moves faster than a platypus or a three-toed sloth. Don't you have any eggs left, either?

Doris: Ugh! Those slimy things!

Herb: Come on, they're not so bad hard-boiled.

Doris: Herb, you know darn well that boiling won't be invented for several thousand years! Get to hunting and gathering you lazy so-and-so. We're hungry!

Our hero leaves his dwelling to go hunt. He has no rifle, no bow-and-arrow, no sling-shot— just a primitive spear, a club, and a handy rock as his weapons. His hunt will take about a week, and he may or may not come back with substantial food. In the meantime, Doris will make small forays from camp to find tubers, nuts, seeds, and insects to tide her family over.

The serious point I'm trying to make (in spite of the lighthearted tone of this "play") is that our hunter-gatherer ancestors didn't eat all that much mainly because food was scarce and methods for obtaining it were primitive. Hunter-gatherers also expended a significant amount of energy while hunting—certainly greater than the calories we use shopping or eating in a restaurant.

The good news is, if you eat along the same guidelines as our hunter-gatherer ancestors, you'll still lose weight, lower your blood cholesterol level, and decrease your risk for cancer.

Calories Count—But Don't Count Calories

Natural forces kept the caloric intake of the hunter-gatherer low. Not only was food scarce, but the available food was low in calories. No agriculture or animal husbandry existed, which meant that there was no fatty meat, milk, cream, or cheese. So hunter-gatherers never had to be concerned with calories, because high-calorie foods were not an option.

In our modern world, we're not so lucky. We're surrounded by fatty, high-calorie foods at every turn. But this doesn't mean that you're going to have to think about the calories in every item of food before you eat it. If you simply stick to the principles of the Evolutionary Diet, your fat intake will be low, which will naturally decrease your total intake of calories.

One of the reasons we're so concerned about fat is that fats have more than twice as many calories by weight as protein or carbohydrates. Fat has nine calories per gram, while protein and carbohydrates have only four calories per gram. So the easiest way to reduce calories (without having to think about the calorie content of everything you eat) is to cut back on your intake of fat.

However, not counting calories doesn't mean we shouldn't be aware of them. High-calorie foods are everywhere, so if we don't consider calories at all, we're likely to get into trouble.

But what exactly is a calorie? It is a measure of energy, just as an inch is a measure of length and a degree is a measure of temperature. A calorie is defined as the amount of energy it takes to raise the temperature of one gram of water one degree centigrade.

Food is energy and has calories. But caloric energy in food is *potential* energy. This energy is expended only in the activities of daily living. The rest of the energy is stored until needed. Calories are stored in the body as glycogen (a type of carbohydrate) and fat. Ideally, the amount of calories you take in is matched by the number of calories used for breathing, walking, exercise, shopping, and even sleeping. But if we take in more calories than we expend, we put on weight.

Isocaloric Diets

How many calories do we need on a daily basis to maintain our ideal weight? Naturally, this number varies from person to person—a lumberjack will need to consume many more calories than a librarian.

In general, a diet in the range of 1,300 to 2,800 calories is sufficient for most people. Of course, that's a big spread. (See Table 2A on the next page for more specific information.) Ideally, we should strive for an isocaloric diet. This means that you're eating the same amount of calories as you're expending on a given day. On an isocaloric diet, your weight will not change.

If you want to lose weight, you will have to either decrease the amount of calories you eat or increase the amount of calories you use, or both. Begin to eat like our hunter-gatherer ancestors, and you will slowly stabilize your weight until you reach the break-even point where the calories you're consuming will be equal to those you are expending.

It's important to know that calories count, but you shouldn't have to count them. If you stick to the Evolutionary Diet, you shouldn't have any problems with excess calories. However, if you're following the principles outlined in this book and you still find that you're not melting down to your ideal weight, you're consuming too many calories. This means that although you're eating low-fat foods, you're probably eating too much of them! That's when you need to give your calorie consumption some thought.

Remember to keep in mind one important food fact: Fat has over twice the number of calories per gram as protein or carbohydrates. This means that the small pat of butter you put on a piece of bread may have more calories in it than the bread itself.

TABLE 2A

NUMBER OF CALORIES THAT MUST BE CONSUMED DAILY TO MAINTAIN YOUR "IDEAL WEIGHT"

(Assuming that 25 percent of your total calories comes from fat, and you work in an office setting)

WOMEN			MEN		
Weight	Calories	Fat (gm.)	Weight	Calories	Fat (gm.)
110	1,300	37	130	1,800	51
120	1,400	40	140	2,000	54
130	1,600	43	150	2,100	58
140	1,700	47	160	2,200	62
150	1,800	50	170	2,400	66
160	1,900	53	180	2,500	70
170	2,000	57	190	2,700	74
180	2,200	60	200	2,800	78

Unfortunately, recent studies show that about half of all Americans are overweight. One of the ways of looking at our weight is by looking at our body mass. Federal guidelines suggest that people should have a body mass index (BMI) of less than 25. The National Health and Nutrition

Examination Survey, conducted on 30,000 people from 1991 to 1994, found that 59 percent of men and 49 percent of women had a BMI over 25. To estimate your BMI, you'll probably need to get out your calculator.

1. Convert your weight into kilograms by multiplying your weight in pounds by 0.45.
2. Figure out your height in inches, and multiply this number by .0254 to convert to meters.
3. Multiply that number (meters) by itself (that is, square it).
4. Divide the result of #3 into the result of #1 (your weight in kilograms).

Don't Forget That There Are Actually Two Cholesterols

Cholesterol is one of the most complicated issues in medicine and health today UNLESS you know a simple fact: There are, for our purposes, two cholesterols: (1) cholesterol that we eat in food, and (2) the cholesterol measured in our blood. They are entirely different.

One of the ways that we have been taken in by the food industry is that we have been subtly led to think of both cholesterols as the same—not only in spelling, but also in importance and relevance.

The truth is, high *blood* cholesterol is bad for you—however, this has been misinterpreted to mean that high cholesterol *foods* are bad for you. Such is not the case. The amount of saturated fat we eat greatly influences our blood cholesterol level, but the cholesterol *in our food is of VERY little importance* in our overall health.

※ ※ ※ ※ ※ ※

Chapter Three

Cancer: Battling the Dark Side of Medicine

I first decided to study oncology in the early '70s, a time when very little was known about the field I was going into. Back then, cancer was a dirty word—the mere mention of which was enough to give most people chills. Unfortunately, the medical community at that time was barely more enlightened than most lay people. Many doctors regarded cancer victims as lepers.

In 1972, amidst the misconceptions and confusion surrounding the disease, I decided to devote my medical career to fighting cancer. I was part of a new, hearty breed of doctors entering medical oncology, an area of medicine that was just coming into existence. My peers and I knew we would face the ultimate medical challenge: We were going to battle the forces of the dark side.

Cancer was and still is a scary diagnosis. But since the '70s, much has been learned about the cause and treatment of this disease. In this chapter, I want to bring you up to speed on what cancer really is, how it is caused, and how it spreads. Most important, I want to tell you how to prevent it.

My reasons for doing so are very personal. Since becoming an oncologist 20 years ago, I have watched thousands of people die from this disease. And as tough as it has been on these patients and their families, I have to admit that it's been tough on me, too. At times, I've been able to do something; other times I've stood by helplessly watching yet another life slip out of my grasp.

It's been a very painful lesson to learn that the best cure for cancer is not a cure at all—it's prevention, risk reduction, and screening. That's why I hope you take to heart the information contained in this book. And maybe you won't slip out of my hands, too.

Oncology 101—Understanding Cancer

You rarely see cancer in children. Why? Because it's a disease that you can't contract overnight. It doesn't happen through one exposure to radiation or by inhaling one whiff of tobacco smoke. It takes decades for the disease to start, years to spread, and months to kill. This gives doctors a lot of time to detect cancer in its earliest form.

So what causes cancer, exactly? We know that it begins with damage to the cell's DNA. This is very serious, because DNA, as you recall, is the blueprint for your body. Just as a blueprint determines how many bathrooms, fireplaces, and doors a house will have, your DNA determines how curly your hair is, how fast your fingernails grow, and how long your arms are.

But DNA doesn't become obsolete once your body is fully grown; DNA controls your body's functions throughout your lifetime. Think of DNA as being the script for your biologic life. On page one, you're told to grow teeth and hair. Around page 13, you go through puberty, and at the end of the play, you simply wear out (assuming you haven't contracted a disease to decrease your lifespan).

DNA also controls the growth of your cells. It tells them whether to grow or grow up. These are two very distinct processes, and when a cell confuses them, cancer may result. *Growing up* has a beginning and an end. It is completed once maturity has been reached. A baby grows up; organs can "grow up" as well. For instance, if a person has a kidney removed, the remaining kidney gets larger—to a point. It "grows up" until it is large enough to compensate for the loss of the other kidney. And then the process ends. The kidney reaches its new size and stops growing.

If you break an arm or a leg, bone begins to grow around the break until the bone has healed. Bone cells know when the task is finished, and they stop growing. But there are also cases when cells and organs normally just grow, such as fingernails and hair. They both continue to grow over the course of your lifetime.

Consider what would happen if the signals got crossed and instead of telling the cell to "grow up," the DNA instructed the cell to just grow. As you've probably already guessed, this is what cancer is: a bunch of mad cells that just grow and grow and grow (without growing up), and in the process, they lose all sense of order. The cells forget their normal function and just concentrate on multiplying.

Cancer is like an automobile production line gone haywire. In the properly functioning production line, raw materials are put together on the assembly line. At the other end, a complete car comes out, fully equipped with four doors, two seats, and a steering wheel. This is "growing up" for a car.

Cancer is like having the production line jam. One of the assemblers quits doing his job, but the conveyor belt keeps on moving. So the cars keeps spilling off the assembly line, but they're missing parts, some of which are vital. Their development has been halted. Cancer makes things grow without growing up; these immature cells simply duplicate and reduplicate themselves.

Cancer formation is a slow process. A cell doesn't go from being normal to cancerous overnight. It takes time for the process to occur. Keep in mind that your body has an amazing ability to protect itself, and it often succeeds in killing off or controlling these dangerous cells before they can pass through each succeeding phase. This is why many women whose Pap smears show premalignant cervical changes will never go on to develop invasive cancer. But if the human body is repeatedly exposed to cancer-causing substances, its defenses are weakened. With each exposure, more genetic damage occurs to normal cells, and they finally lose all of the niceties of good behavior and become cancer cells that grow, invade, duplicate themselves, and kill.

Phases of Cancer

In order for cancer to "succeed," it must spread, but as I've already explained, this is not an instantaneous process. Growing and duplicating is only the first step. Once that occurs, cancer must pass through several other stages:

1. Cancer cells (just like any other cells) require oxygen and food. They get this nutrition from the blood, so in order to survive, cancer cells coax blood vessels to grow toward them. (Of interesting note: Researchers are currently testing drugs that may stop cancer at this early phase.)

2. After they're well fed, cancer cells start to develop the ability to spread. The strongest ones acquire the ability to leave "home" and begin traveling through the body.

3. These maverick cells squeeze themselves out of the confines of the organ and get into the blood and lymph vessels.

4. In the bloodstream and lymph channels, they face even greater challenges. The bloodstream is a noxious environment, and the cancer cells, which really don't belong there, must have acquired enough genetic know-how to protect themselves against the body's own defenses. In the bloodstream, there are "police" who destroy strangers and trespassers on sight, but the heartiest cancer cells can make cloaking devices that render them invisible.

5. Now the cancer cells must land someplace, but this too is not a random process. Certain cancers preferentially spread to certain organs. There has to be a "fit" between the cancer cell and its landing field. Depending on the type of cancer, cells may spread to the kidneys, the bones, the lungs, or any other organ they are programmed to invade. Once cancer cells invade an organ, they form growing colonies of cancer cells called metastases.

6. As these cancer cells grow, they take up room and eventually interfere with the functioning of the organ in which they are residing. For instance, cancer cells in the bone begin replacing normal bone tissue. Eventually, this causes bones to weaken and fracture.

7. Once cancer has found a place to settle and grow, the process begins all over again. New cancer cells grow, acquire a blood supply, squeeze their way into blood and lymph vessels, travel through the bloodstream, and so on.

8. Finally, there are so many cancer cells that the body is overwhelmed.

Cancer-Causing Agents

I've already explained that cancer is the process of cumulative genetic change, but what mechanisms bring this about?

One cause is hormonal changes in the body. The reduction or increase of hormones is (at least partly) to blame for breast, prostate, and ovarian cancer. The reason for this, in oversimplified terms, is that the more time a cell spends dividing, the more errors it can make. And hormones can make a cell divide or not, depending on the hormone and the exact situation.

Many chemical agents have also been linked with cancer. Tobacco smoke, nickel, wood dust, petroleum products, alcohol, and vinyl chloride are just a few examples. (See Table 3A on the next page.) Many of these chemicals combine with parts of the DNA, causing gene activations or inactivations, which make the DNA less able to carry out its functions.

One exposure to a cancer-promoting substance is probably not enough to start most malignancies. There has to be continual damage over a period of years before enough errors are made by the DNA to affect its normal function. That is why smokers get cancer after years of smoking, printers get cancer after years of exposure to petroleum-based inks, and shoe repairmen get cancer after years of working with polish and leather dust.

Radiation is another dangerous carcinogen. It acts like a molecular scissors, cutting the strands of DNA. However, for many years, we were not fully aware of the hazards of radioactive substances.

The most famous story of radiation-induced cancer is the saga of the luminous watches. Decades ago, radium was used to make watches glow in the dark. Workers in the factories would paint the radium onto the watches by hand, using tiny paintbrushes. To get a fine tip, they would lick the end of the paintbrush, which caused them to ingest significant amounts of this radioactive element. Years later, most of these workers came down with fatal bone and bone marrow cancers.

TABLE 3A

OCCUPATIONAL EXPOSURE TO CANCER-CAUSING AGENTS IN THE WORKPLACE

Agent	Type of Exposure	Type of Cancer
Alcohol	Manufacturing	Nasal, sinus
Aluminum	Manufacturing	Lung
Analine dyes	Dye manufacturing	Bladder
Arsenic	Mining, pesticides	Lung, skin, liver
Asbestos	Plumbing, insulation	Lung, stomach
Benzene	Leather, petroleum	Leukemia
Benzidine	Various manufacturing	Bladder
Bis-chloromethyl ether	Resins	Lung
Cadmium	Batteries	Prostate
Chromium	Pigment manufacturing	Lung
Isopropyl alcohol	Alcohol manufacturing	Sinus
Leather industry	Manufacturing and repair	Nasal, bladder
Nickel dust	Refining	Lung, nasal
Pesticides	Application	Lung, lymphoma
Polycyclic hydrocarbons	Petroleum industry	Lung, skin
Radiation	Mining	Most sites
UV light	Farming/Fishing industries	Skin
Vinyl chloride	Polyvinyl chloride	Liver
Wood dust	Manufacturing	Nasal

Viruses are another cause of cancer. They get into cells and interfere with the working of DNA until a cancer is eventually produced. A good example of this is cancer of the cervix. It is now felt that this cancer is caused by the infection of papilloma viruses that can be picked up during normal, unprotected intercourse.

You Don't Have to Get Cancer

Nearly everyone is afraid of getting cancer. Part of this fear stems from lack of understanding, yet part of this fear is justified. *The good (and amazing!) news is that a healthy diet seems to have a preventative effect—even among people who have been exposed to cancer-causing substances.* Eating a diet similar to that of our Cro-Magnon ancestors is among the best ways to avoid this life-threatening disease.

I continue to read statistics of isolated tribes that have no appreciable rates of cancer. And I constantly come across findings that people living on similar diets (such as Seventh Day Adventists, Mormons, and vegetarians) have reduced rates for most cancers when compared with the rest of the population. The connection between diet and disease is clear, as is the use of diet to help reduce risk.

As you continue through this book, you'll learn more about how to eat correctly to help protect yourself from this potentially fatal disease. In chapter eleven, I'll also tell you about some of the great progress that has been made in the treatment and early diagnosis of cancer.

❋ ❋ ❋ ❋ ❋ ❋

Chapter Four

Hunting, Anyone?

For us humans, the best sources of protein are wild animals. They're low in overall fat, low in saturated fat and, unlike commercially raised livestock, they aren't filled with chemicals or added hormones. The problem is, it's tough for the modern grocery shopper to go hunting. The mastodon population is down, deer are hard to find in cities and suburbs, and foraging around for small rodents isn't really an option. So what's a modern-day Cro-Magnon to do?

Don't worry. You're not going to have to forego evolutionary eating just because you can't get fresh or frozen giraffe, lion, or eland at your local supermarket. There are plenty of sources of protein that are nutritious, low in fat, and easy to find.

Wild Game Versus Domesticated Meats

Just as humans suffer from the fruits of our modern civilization, animals also suffer when we impose our civilization on them. When animals are allowed to graze, and to eat what's found in their natural environments, they're healthy and their bodies are low in fat. But when animals are cooped up and fed foods that they've never even seen before, their bodies degenerate in the same way that ours do.

One of the most extreme examples of this is Japanese Kobe beef. These cattle are fed a high-fat diet (including beer!) and live in stalls where they never get any exercise. (But they do get massaged by their keepers. Must be rough!) The result is a beef no self-respecting steer would be proud of. And this unhealthful delicacy sells for around $130 a pound in the U.S.!

Farm-raised cattle live in very similar circumstances (they're fattened up in feed lots, but without the beer) and, in general, this meat is not much healthier for you. Even lean ground beef is 61 percent fat in terms of calories (even though it says 15 percent fat on the label—we'll talk more about deceptive meat-labeling practices later in this chapter).

What about free-range meat? Although roaming free certainly makes life more pleasant for the animals, it doesn't make the meat much healthier. Farmers take into account the fact that these animals are getting exercise, so they're fattened up with a high-fat diet in feed lots before slaughter.

At the other end of the spectrum, we find wild game. In their natural environments, these animals have little fat in their meat because they're eating a low-fat diet and roaming free. For example, wild boar has less than half the fat of its domesticated counterpart. Likewise, bison has nearly half the fat content of farm-raised cattle.

TABLE 4A

DIFFERENT FAT CONTENTS IN WILD VS. DOMESTIC MEAT*

Beef 3 oz.	Calories	Fat (gm.)	Saturated Fat (gm.)
Farm-raised (brisket)	206	10.9	3.9
Wild bison	122	2.1	0.8
Pork 3 oz.			
Spareribs (lean)	337	25.8	10.0
Wild boar	136	3.7	1.1

* Sources for table data are listed at the end of the chapter.

Beware of Misleading Labels

I've already explained that you should aim to get no more than 25 percent of your calories from fat. "Great," you say. "Then I should be able to eat all the beef I want because the label tells me that it's only 17 percent fat."

If only this were the case. That 17 percent may sound good, but this number is misleading because it's calculated by weight. (In other words, roughly every five pounds of meat will include almost a pound of fat.) Counting fat as a function of weight rather than calories is a serious biologic error, because metabolically the body responds to calories. You don't go on a diet of "two pounds" of food a day. And you know that a pound of grapes is not the same as a pound of cheese. You're concerned with how many calories an item contains, not how much it weighs.

So why do meat companies express fat content this way? For the simple reason that 17 percent fat sounds a lot better for you than 61 percent. Unfortunately, it doesn't make the meat any healthier.

Take a look at some comparisons of fat content by weight and by calories:

TABLE 4B

PERCENT FAT CONTENT OF BEEF: WEIGHT VS. CALORIES*

Meat	% Fat by Weight	% Fat by Calories
Extra lean ground beef	16	58
Lean ground beef	18	61
Regular ground beef	21	66

* Sources for table data are listed at the end of the chapter.

"Bad Meats" Versus "Good Meats"

All meat contains about the same amount of protein, so when we compare healthy and unhealthy meats, we're really looking at two things:

1. The total amount of fat
2. The amount of saturated fat

Remember, we're concerned with keeping the total fat content of our diets at less than 25 percent, and we want to eat as little saturated fat as possible. Given these limitations, there are certain meats that you should avoid altogether:

1. **Most domesticated red meat.** This meat is not only high in fat, but a whopping percentage of the fat is saturated. Take a look at some of these numbers:

TABLE 4C

BEEF FAT CONTENT AND SATURATED FAT CONTENT AS A PERCENTAGE OF TOTAL CALORIES*

Meat	% Fat Content	% Saturated Fat
Lean ground beef	61	24
Corned beef	54	22
Chuck blade roast	71	30
Beef shortribs	80	34

* Sources for table data are listed at the end of the chapter.

2. **Pork and lamb.** Saying that a pork chop may be better for your health than a hamburger is like saying that playing Russian Roulette with .22 bullets are safer for you than .45s. Pork in general is lower in fat and saturated fat than red meat, but the fat content is still way out of the healthful range

However, there is one exception to the rule that pork is bad for you. Pork truly can be the "other white meat" in one instance: The tenderloin of pork is naturally lean. When well trimmed and roasted or grilled, it can be as low as 26 percent calories from fat. For this reason, we have included several pork tenderloin recipes in this book.

TABLE 4D

FAT CONTENT/SATURATED FAT CONTENT OF OTHER MEATS AS A PERCENTAGE OF TOTAL CALORIES*

Meat	% Fat Content	% Saturated Fat
Picnic ham (fat in)	67	24
Bacon, broiled	78	27
Bacon, uncooked	93	35
Leg of lamb (fat in)	61	34
Trimmed leg of lamb	34 **	19
Lamb chop (fat in)	74	41
Trimmed lamb chop	36 **	21

* Sources for table data are listed at the end of the chapter.

**Look at what a difference trimming can make! Unfortunately, 34 percent and 36 percent fat is still a bit too high to be eating even trimmed lamb on a regular basis.*

3. **Processed meats.** It's easy to see how Americans get a huge portion of their fat from processed meats: Most of them contain 70 to 80 percent fat (in terms of total calories). Even some turkey substitutes for sausages are barely more healthful than their beef/pork counterparts because companies add moisture to these products by adding fat.

TABLE 4E

FAT CONTENT/SATURATED FAT CONTENT OF PROCESSED MEATS AS A PERCENTAGE OF TOTAL CALORIES*

Meat	% Fat Content	% Saturated Fat
Beef bologna	83	35
Bratwurst	77	28
Hot dog	82	35
Turkey hot dog	73	24
Salami (beef)	82	36
Salami (dry pork)	75	26
Turkey salami	64	19
Pastrami	75	27

Enough about what you *can't* eat; let's move on to the meats you *can* eat. There are plenty of sources of protein that are delicious and good for you. We'll start by talking about the healthiest: shellfish and fish.

1. **Shellfish and fish**. Shellfish and fish (which are most often wild) are wonderful foods. Even fish with the highest fat content (those that live in cold water and require fat as insulation to keep them warm) are relatively low in fat, and most of this fat is unsaturated. They also contain large quantities of the health-promoting fish oil Eicasopentanoic Acid (EPA)—more about this in chapter eight.

    If fish earn silver stars in the category of healthy eating, shellfish earn gold ones. I would go as far as to say that shrimp, oysters, lobsters, and crab are *ideal foods*. They're wonderful sources of protein that contain less than 10 percent saturated fat.

    Try to make shellfish or fish your main sources of protein, and supplement them occasionally with poultry and wild game.

TABLE 4F

FAT CONTENT/SATURATED FAT CONTENT OF SHELLFISH AND FISH AS A PERCENTAGE OF TOTAL CALORIES

Fish (Raw)	% Fat	% Saturated Fat
Abalone	6	1
Crayfish	11	2
Clams	11	1
Shrimp	15	3
Oysters, Pacific	26	5
Mussels	23	5
Crab, Dungeness	10	1
Lobster	9	trace
Octopus	12	3
Squid	14	3
Scallops	10	2
Sea Bass, striped	22	4
Snapper	12	2

Fish (Raw)	% Fat	% Saturated Fat
Monkfish	18	trace
Halibut	19	3
Tuna, yellowfin	8	2
Whitefish	39	6
Whitefish, smoked	8	2
Swordfish	30	8
Shark	31	6
Salmon, Coho	37	7

*Sources for table data are listed at the end of the chapter.

2. **Poultry.** Technically, poultry is domesticated meat, but it's low in fat and saturated fat, so it's allowed on the Evolutionary Diet. Eat poultry several times a week to add variety to your meals, but keep the following tips in mind:

Eat more white meat than dark. White meat is much lower in fat than dark meat.

Take off the skin. Taking off the skin cuts the fat calories in half! If you leave it on while cooking to add flavor and retain moisture, you will be adding some fat calories to the meat, but fewer than if you eat the skin. It's a good compromise when eating plain chicken without a sauce.

TABLE 4G

POULTRY CALORIES AND FAT CONTENT AS A PERCENTAGE OF TOTAL CALORIES*

Turkey 3½ oz.	Calories	% Fat Content
White meat with skin	197	40
White meat without skin	157	18
Dark meat with skin	221	47
Dark meat without skin	187	35

Chicken 3½ oz.	Calories	% Fat Content
White meat with skin	222	44
White meat without skin	173	23
Dark meat with skin	253	56
Dark meat without skin	205	43

*Sources for table data are listed at the end of the chapter.

3. **Wild game.** Wild game is getting easier to find every day. The other day at the entrance to my neighborhood grocery store, I saw a sign advertising "Ostrich, the Healthy Red Meat." Not only does my market carry ostrich burgers, ostrich franks, and ostrich steak, I can also buy buffalo, bison, kangaroo, and venison there. The truth is, ostrich is farm raised now, and thus not wild, but we include it in the "wild" category because it is very low in fat.

    I live in a large city where markets carry nondomesticated meats. If you live out in the country, wild game, a wonderful low-fat source of protein, is generally easier to get.

    You can also order wild game from one of the suppliers listed in Appendix II at the back of this book. Or talk to your local butcher. Most will be happy to provide you with any type of meat you request.

TABLE 4H

FAT CALORIES OF WILD MEAT AS A PERCENTAGE OF TOTAL CALORIES

Type of Wild Meat	% Fat Calories
Pheasant without skin, raw	24
Venison	18
Elk	12
Moose	7
Frogs' legs	4
Ostrich	18

* Sources for table data are listed at the end of the chapter.

4. **Other sources of protein.** Do you think that the only way to get your protein is to consume something that moves? If so, I understand; I used to believe the same thing. But it's not true! Some of the most flavorful and nutritious protein comes in the form of beans, peas, and lentils (see Table 4I). For example, a serving of white beans has 120 calories but zero percent fat calories! Make these and other legumes part of your meals on a regular basis.

TABLE 4I

LOW-FAT SOURCES OF PROTEIN

Item	% Fat Calories	% Protein Calories
Black beans	4	28
Broccoli	10	56
Cauliflower	1	33
Egg whites	0	100
Green peas	5	27
Green beans	0	24
Lentils	3	33
Nonfat cottage cheese	0	74
Nonfat yogurt	0	44

Preparing Meats

Now that you know what types of meat to eat, let me give you some final tips to reduce the fat content even further.

1. **Have your meat trimmed.** Trimming your meat reduces the amount of fat you'll end up eating. This is easy enough to do because in wild animals, fat is on the outside of the meat. (In domesticated animals, it's marbled, which means it grows between the muscle fibers.)

2. **Try to grill, pan roast, or barbecue.** These methods of cooking poultry and wild game allow most of the remaining fat to drip off, making the meat healthier and lower in calories.

3. **Before eating poultry, be sure to take off the skin.** Remove the skin, and you'll cut the fat calories almost in half.

4. **Separate the fat from pan juices.** If you want to cook with pan juices, remove the fat first by spooning it off or by using a separator.

5. **Never bread anything.** Breading acts like a sponge for fat. Look at what breading does to the fat content of otherwise healthy meats:

TABLE 4J

FAT CALORIES FOR COOKED VS. BREADED MEATS AS A PERCENTAGE OF TOTAL CALORIES*

Meat	% Cooked	% Breaded and Fried
Catfish	32	52
Oysters	26	57
Chicken	23	45

*Sources for table data are listed at the end of the chapter.

Go On, Be Daring!

When it comes to eating meat, you can stick to seafood, poultry, and an occasional piece of *very* lean red meat, and you'll do just fine—you'll lower your cholesterol and avoid many life-threatening diseases.

But if you want to add variety to your diet, don't be afraid to be adventurous. Walk out of that fish and chicken aisle and step into the wild. Try eating bison, buffalo, or ostrich. Or really live on the edge and sample frogs' legs, eel, or snail.

If you love to eat as much as I do, you'll want to start cooking foods that your friends may never even have heard of, and then invite them over to dinner. I guarantee that your friends will want to start living on the culinary frontier right along with you.

❈ ❈ ❈

Chapter Four Table Data Derived from the Following Sources:

Bowes and Church's Food Values of Portions Commonly Used, Sixteenth Edition, Revised by Jean A. T. Rennington, Ph.D., R.D.; J.B. Lippincott Company, Philadelphia, 1994.

Composition of Foods: Lamb, Veal & Game Products. Agricultural Handbook, USDA, 1989.

Composition of Foods: Finfish and Shellfish Products. Agricultural Handbook, USDA, 1989.

Prevention Magazine's Complete Nutrition Reference Handbook. Mark Bricklin, Rodale Press, Emmaus, PA, 1992.

※ ※ ※ ※ ※ ※

Chapter Five

Cro-Magnons Didn't Eat Candy Bars

I magine the way the world looked 30,000 years ago. There was no Ben and Jerry's ice cream, no Bakers Square pies, no Hershey bars, and no New York cheesecake. (In fact, there wasn't even a New York!)

What the world was full of was a lot of tubers (starchy vegetables such as potatoes and yams), beans, fruits, and nuts. This is how Cro-Magnons got the bulk of their carbohydrates, and it's the same way we should be eating.

Unfortunately, most of us get our carbohydrates from processed foods, which have little nutritional value and are full of fat. We also eat far too many sweets.

In this chapter, I'll provide you with some healthy sources for getting energy-filled foods. I'll also explain the surprising role refined sugar may play in promoting hardening of the arteries. But first, a few words about carbohydrates....

Understanding Carbohydrates

Carbohydrates and sugars are closely related. Both provide your body with energy, but because sugar is digested much more easily, it gives your body a quick rush. Carbohydrates (which are actually chains of sugar molecules strung together) are broken down more slowly. Your body uses what's needed and stores the rest in the form of glycogen.

When the body needs additional energy, it turns to its glycogen reserves. This is the reason that runners "carb load." The night before a marathon, they eat lots of starches so that during the race, when they need more energy, their bodies will break down glycogen for this purpose (rather than breaking down fat or protein, which can result in unwanted physical consequences).

Since carbohydrates and sugars both provide the body with energy, is eating sugar cubes just as good as eating potatoes? As you intuitively know, the answer is no. If you were to eat only sugar, you'd be depriving your body of the other nutritional benefits (such as fiber and vitamins) that are found in carbohydrate-rich foods. This doesn't mean you can't have an occasional spoonful of sugar in your coffee; it's just that large quantities of sugar consumed over a period of time can have serious effects on your health. I'll tell you more about that later in the chapter.

❖ ❖ ❖

Your cells consist of three main components: carbohydrates, protein, and fat (with a little water and minerals thrown in). Because they form such an important part of your body's makeup, carbohydrates should also comprise a large part of what you eat.

Interestingly enough, in some countries such as Greece and Italy, where carbohydrates are a very important part of people's diets, rates of cancer and heart disease are substantially lower than in the United States. The Italians eat just as much sugar as we do, but they also eat about three times as much fresh fruit and twice as many vegetables. Similarly, the average person in Greece eats twice as much fruit and about 30 times more legumes! Even though the Greeks eat about the same amount of fat as most Americans, their rate of coronary heart disease is a fraction of ours, and their rates of breast and colon cancer are about a third of ours.

TABLE 5A

COMPARATIVE DIETARY CONSUMPTION:
U.S. VS. ITALY

The following chart depicts the amount of each food category consumed
per person/per year in Italy and the United States.

CATEGORY	PER CAPITA: AMERICA	PER CAPITA: ITALY
Pasta	18.4 lbs.	55.1 lbs.
Olive oil	<0.1 gal.	3.0 gal.
Wine	2.0 gal.	18.4 gal.
Tomato products	70.3 lbs.	139.0 lbs.
Sugar	64.0 lbs.	52.2 lbs.
Coffee	10.2 lbs.	11.2 lbs.
Bread	50.5 lbs.	139.0 lbs.
Rice	17.0 lbs.	11.0 lbs.
Fresh fruit	89.0 lbs.	286.0 lbs.
Pork	64.5 lbs.	59.0 lbs.
Beef	95.1 lbs.	57.6 lbs.
Chicken	73.4 lbs.	42.0 lbs.
Veal	1.2 lbs.	3.9 lbs.
Fish	14.8 lbs.	25.7 lbs.
Milk	221.6 lbs.	174.6 lbs.
Butter	4.4 lbs.	4.4 lbs.
Eggs	30.2 lbs.	24.2 lbs.
Cheeses	24.7 lbs.	35.4 lbs.

Each number represents the most recent year that a figure for consumption was calculated. All figures
for Italy converted from kg. Figures for meats are carcass weights as opposed to retail weights.
Sources: U.S. Department of Agriculture; Italian Trade Commission; Bertolli, Inc.; U.S. Department
of Commerce; National Pasta Association; National Restaurant Association

Carbohydrates are energy foods, and they should form the bulk of your
diet. About 50 percent of your calories (the same amount that our hunter-
gatherer ancestors consumed) will come from this source if you follow the
Evolutionary Diet plan.

Carbohydrates come in a variety of forms. They're found in vegetables, grains, nuts, and beans. Fruit also contains carbohydrates but in a slightly different form. The sweeter a carbohydrate source is, the more simple carbohydrates (that is, sugars) it will have.

Baked Goods

Obviously, the art and science of baking and pastry making was not known 30,000 years ago. Although our Cro-Magnon ancestors may have gathered some grain, they lacked the knowledge of how to grind this grain into flour, and they certainly had no methods for baking bread.

So where do baked goods fit in with evolutionary eating? In general, they don't (although eating a limited amount of some breads, preferably whole grain bread, is okay). Most baked goods (including many pastries, croissants, pies, and cakes) are high in sugar and/or fat. Even that healthy-sounding bran muffin may be filled with coconut or palm oil. And many baking mixes contain high amounts of fat and salt. The only way to be sure is to read the labels.

Graham crackers are a notable exception. With some searching, you may be able to find some that are less than 20 percent fat. (Keep in mind, however, that graham crackers do contain a good deal of sugar.) Also, rice wafers contain no fat and very little sodium (but it's hard to make a sandwich with them). Another problem with baked goods is that many of them contain appreciable amounts of salt. However, you can find low-sodium bread that doesn't taste too bad.

What about the difference between white and whole wheat flours? In general, the distinction is similar to that between refined and "natural" sugars. Whole wheat breads provide your body with the same amount of carbohydrates as white breads; however, whole wheat has more nutrients and fiber. You're best off trying to limit your intake of baked goods, while keeping in mind that whole grains provide more nutrients than their refined counterparts.

Sugars and Insulin

When you eat sugar, your body produces insulin. Insulin is a very helpful molecule that allows us to metabolize sugar, but it also has a very unfortunate side effect: There seems to be a relationship between higher blood levels of insulin and the development of hardening of the arteries.

If you recall, arteriosclerosis begins with damage to the inside lining of the arteries. In addition to saturated fat, insulin can be one of the causes of this injury.

In one significant and interesting study, researchers took blood samples from a group of healthy people. Years later, investigators re-examined these blood specimens and found that the subjects who went on to have heart attacks had slightly higher insulin levels than those who didn't. This study has been repeated several times in different parts of the world with similar results.

Besides its potential to exacerbate hardening of the arteries, refined sugar gives the body a jolt that is not natural. Tachycardia (a high heart rate) and the low blood sugar that follows the initial rush are unwelcome effects. These dramatic ups and downs are especially likely to happen when you eat a food high in sugar (such as a candy bar) on an empty stomach.

But what about honey, molasses, maple syrup, and fructose? Are these sugars better for you than refined sugar? The answer depends on what is meant by "better for you."

Your body processes these "natural" sugars in the same way it metabolizes refined sugar. In other words, you get a rapid energy rush, and insulin is produced. In that sense, they're no healthier for you than refined sugars. However, natural sugars contain other nutrients that refined sugars lack (for instance, molasses is rich in iron, calcium, and potassium).

On the whole, you're better off cutting your intake of sweets in general instead of worrying about what form of sugar you're eating.

※ ※ ※ ※ ※ ※

Chapter Six

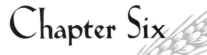

Uh-Oh,
Milk Is Full of Fat!

"Drink your milk. It's full of calcium. Milk makes strong bones and healthy teeth." Your mother thought she was giving you good advice—the only problem was, your mother wasn't a Cro-Magnon. No self-respecting Cro-Mag mom would ever tell her kids to drink their milk. (In fact, Cro-Magnon mothers didn't tell their kids much of anything, since language consisted of a few rudimentary grunts and gestures, but...details, details!)

Our Cro-Magnon ancestors lived just fine (and very healthily!) without drinking milk as adults. Once they had been weaned, hunter-gatherers never again ate dairy foods in any form. In fact, modern humans are the only species on the face of the earth that continues the practice of drinking milk past early childhood. Dolphins are weaned, and raccoons are, too; even baby cows stop drinking the milk that we keep putting into our bodies as adults. Think about that, and you'll get an intuitive sense of how "unnatural" drinking milk truly is.

The fact is, dairy foods are our own worst health enemies. In this chapter, I'll show you how to eliminate them from your diet without eliminating the calcium that is essential for strong bones and healthy teeth.

Dairy Foods

Dairy products have more calories from fat than many other "natural" foods. Worse yet, most of this fat is saturated (that is, the artery-clogging kind). Cow's milk gets 51 percent of its calories from fat. And milk from other species is no better. Goat's milk gets almost 58 percent of its calories from fat. Human milk (would you believe?!) is almost 60 percent fat. (We'll talk more about infant nutrition later.)

Regular yogurt is similar to milk: 48 percent of its calories come from fat. Cheese is even worse. Most of the tastier, smellier cheeses (such as blue cheese) contain about 75 percent fat, almost all of which is saturated. Take a look at a few of these numbers:

TABLE 6A

FAT CONTENT OF CHEESE AS A PERCENTAGE OF TOTAL CALORIES*

Cheese	% Fat
Blue	74
Brie	75
Gouda	70
Swiss	66
Cheddar	74
Monterey jack	73
Parmesan	59
Velveeta sharp	65

* Sources for table data listed at the end of chapter four.

As high in fat as cheese is, butter is even worse. Butter is pure fat—that's 100 percent. And it's mostly saturated fat.

Knowing how bad for you these foods are, what should you do? Try to avoid dairy foods in their "natural" (that is, regular fat) form completely. On the next page, I'll give you some advice on eating nonfat dairy foods and other sources of calcium.

The Importance of Calcium

Calcium is an essential part of a healthy diet—especially for women. My mother has served as a painful firsthand reminder of this fact. She was a follower of Carlton Fredericks, a health guru of the '30s. Most of Fredericks' advice was very good. He was a man ahead of the traditional nutritional wisdom of his time. As a kid, the thing I remember most was that he advocated putting wheat germ on everything. I had wheat germ steak, wheat germ salad, and wheat germ yogurt.

But the most interesting thing about Fredericks was his claim that if you ate his diet, you'd live to be 100. Sure enough, my mother is now almost 90. But Fredericks' diet neglected one thing: It was low in calcium and, unfortunately, osteoporosis was the one illness that was going to affect my mother. Healthy in every other way, my mother suffers from that ailment. She is bent like a pretzel, walking is almost impossible, and her quality of life is poor.

I tell you my mother's story to emphasize the importance of consuming enough calcium, especially for women.

❈ ❈ ❈

One way of ensuring that you're getting all the calcium your body needs is by eating nonfat dairy foods. Both nonfat milk and nonfat yogurt contain NO FAT. However, a word of caution: Nonfat dairy foods are okay, but low-fat ones are not! Even low-fat dairy foods are too high in fat to be considered part of the Evolutionary Diet. Although their fat percentages may look okay, the majority of the fat is in the saturated form. Low-fat milk is 23 percent fat by calories.

What about reduced-fat cheeses? Unfortunately, there are really few nonfat alternatives to most cheeses. I have seen cheeses that claim to be low in fat, but the difference in fat between them and their regular counterparts is minor. I picked up one brand of cream cheese and found that the "light" variety got 81 percent of its calories from fat. (The regular cream cheese had 84 percent fat—not a significant difference.)

Dry curd cottage cheese is the only cheese regularly available that is truly low-fat. It contains only about 4 percent fat. Other cheeses that are becoming available in the nonfat variety are cottage cheese, ricotta, and cream cheese.

Other Sources of Calcium

Adults need anywhere from 800 to 2,000 mg. of calcium per day, depending on their age, gender, and other factors. The easiest and best way to ingest that amount is, naturally, from food. In addition to nonfat dairy products, the following foods serve as excellent calcium sources:

- Calcium-fortified orange juice
- Broccoli
- Canned sardines and salmon with bones
- Fortified cereals
- Greens—turnips, mustard, kale, Swiss chard, bok choy, spinach
- Dried beans
- Figs
- Oranges

If you wish to supplement your diet with calcium pills, you should first have a discussion with your doctor. I generally recommend 1,500 mg. per day.

※ ※ ※ ※ ※ ※

Chapter Seven

Healthy Diets Begin in the Womb

Go into any school cafeteria, and you'll see the kinds of foods children in America are growing up on today: whole milk, burgers, french fries, and other fat-filled items. And school lunches are only the tip of the problem. Childhood nutrition is deficient almost from the moment of conception. A mother's poor eating habits directly affect the health of her unborn child. After birth, the high-fat formulas and processed foods most infants are fed contribute to an equally deficient diet.

Heart Disease and Cancer Begin at an Early Age

Kids are eating the same way that most Americans do; sadly enough, this means that they're starting down the road to illness at a very early age. Studies have shown that young adults, children, and even infants show early signs of hardening of the arteries. Once the process starts, it continues to worsen for the rest of a person's life—unless nutritional changes are made. Luckily, the rate of progression can be slowed down or halted entirely by following the principles of the Evolutionary Diet.

A growing fetus has only one source for food: Nutrients in its mother's blood. If a high-fat, high-saturated fat diet is eaten during pregnancy, it means that it will be passed on to the baby (who has nothing else to eat and can't step out to the local salad bar). Very little research has been done on this important issue; however, the Evolutionary Diet is health-promoting at any age, and the earlier it begins, the better the consequences will be.

While pregnant and nursing, mothers should partake of the Evolutionary Diet, with special emphasis on foods containing vitamin E, including fish and fish oils. When the child is ready for solid food, he or she should remain on the Evolutionary Diet with special emphasis on foods containing essential fatty acids, especially fish and fish oils (see Table 8A on page 67).

After birth, a similar problem occurs: Mother's milk, which the infant is completely dependent upon for its nutrition, is a mirror of what the mother is eating. (I'll talk about babies fed on formula in the next section.) Studies in the United States have shown that women eating a low-fat diet have much less harmful fat in their milk than women eating a "regular" diet. However, the good fats—the ones that are essential for the development of the brain—are not diminished on a low-fat diet. This means that mother's milk is protected to some degree from the dietary *deficiencies* of the mother. Yet the composition of a mother's milk is not protected from the dietary *excesses* of the mother. A lactating woman eating a diet high in saturated fat will be passing these nonessential and harmful fats to her nursing child. The composition of mother's milk in Central American countries (where fat intake is lower) is lower in fats than the composition of the average mother's milk in the United States. However, both contain essential fatty acids necessary for growth and development of the brain and nervous system.

Biologically, there is no need for a woman to produce a high-in-saturated-fat breast milk for her nursing infant. In fact, when a mother eats a high-fat diet, she is not only putting herself at risk for all the diseases that we have discussed, she is also putting her child at risk and initiating early blood vessel damage.

What continues to amaze me is that nursing mothers are warned by their doctors against eating certain foods such as garlic and chocolate (that may not agree with a nursing baby), yet rarely are pregnant women told anything about the effects of a diet high in saturated fat. In fact, when weaned, most infants are only weaned halfway. After weaning, milk is completely unnecessary for normal human growth and development. In spite of this fact, once we have weaned our children from their mother's milk, we then begin feeding them cow's milk. This practice of drinking milk usually continues into adulthood.

Unfortunately, whole dairy products are some of our worst health enemies. Half of their calories come from fat, and most of this fat is saturated. The necessary calcium they provide can easily be obtained from other natural sources or tablets. Furthermore, the composition of cow's milk itself is quite different from human milk. Cow's milk is designed to help a calf grow up to become a mature cow and doesn't have much relevance in helping a human baby grow into a thinking organism. A mother who wants her child to grow up healthy might consider a longer period of breast-feeding before weaning. Yet, when weaning occurs, there need not be any more milk in the diet.

A Formula for Poor Nutrition

Ten years ago, I did some research on the fat content of various brands of infant formula. I went to the grocery store and compared nutritional labels and was disturbed to find that most of them contained 45 percent fat (in terms of calories). As the years went by and nutritional information was promoted and advocated, I thought that things would improve. Amazingly, even today, most infant formulas made by the giant companies that we all know contain 45 to 50 percent fat.

The problem with infant formula is that it has been modeled after mother's milk—it has about the same fat content as the milk produced by a woman eating the typical American diet of at least 35 to 45 percent fat. This is pretty depressing news. It means that even if a mother wants to feed her child a low-fat diet and is eating one herself, there are few options in the marketplace to find truly low-fat formulas.

Prepared baby foods are sometimes no better. Meat products can be especially high in fat. Below are some of the fat contents on the nutritional labels of baby foods I found in our local supermarket in 1996.

TABLE 7A

FAT CONTENT OF PREPARED BABY FOOD AS A PERCENTAGE OF TOTAL CALORIES

Baby Food	% Fat Content
Spaghetti and beef	55
Meat sticks	63
Chicken sticks	54
Turkey	58
Lamb	38
Chicken puree	45

The list goes on and on. Even many soy-based baby products are similarly high in fat. However, other baby foods are fine, especially those containing fruits and/or vegetables. I found one brand of sweet potato and turkey that had only 18 percent fat and a combination of pears and chicken that had only 20 percent fat. Pure vegetable purees are often even lower. The message, of course, is read the labels before you buy.

Fat Is an Acquired Taste

In modern-day America, we develop the taste for fat at a very early age. The average fetus gets high-fat food, the average infant gets high-fat food, and the average child eats a high-fat diet. By the time children grow into adults, they have already been programmed in the ways of poor nutrition and feel deprived without a "sack of fat" from the local fast-food restaurant.

Luckily, most people lose their taste for fat once they begin changing their eating habits. After my wife, Kathye, began following the Evolutionary Diet plan, she found that eating a high-fat meal such as a Porterhouse steak made her feel uncomfortably full and lethargic. Now she prefers the taste of lighter foods such as grilled fish and lobster.

Essential Fatty Acids for Children

Keeping children healthy isn't always easy. There are even some scientists and nutritionists who argue that a high-fat diet in childhood and infancy is, in fact, healthy. They argue that certain essential fatty acids that help make up the brain can only be obtained through food. A lack of these fats leads to poor brain development and a decreased ability to think.

Of course, there are some fats that we need for growth and development of the brain and the nervous system. And some of these fats are unable to be manufactured in our bodies. These are the "essential fatty acids." Remember: While pregnant and nursing, a woman should eat essential fatty acids and supplement them for her growing child. A diet high in saturated fat is *not* recommended. Giving helpless babies what is known to be bad for adults is shortsighted and dangerous.

Children need to be taught the benefits of healthy nutrition while they are young. And mothers need to eat well while they're pregnant and breast-feeding. Only in this way can we improve the lot of the next generation and begin to achieve health and wellness in our modern civilization.

❊ ❊ ❊ ❊ ❊ ❊

Chapter Eight

Vitamins, Megavitamins, and Other Health Surprises

Take a walk down the vitamin aisle of your grocery or health food store, and you're bound to be overwhelmed. Not only will you find dozens of different types of vitamins and minerals, you'll have to decide between numerous brands, combinations, additives, and doses.

Given the huge variety of supplements available and the amount of money to be made selling them, it's no wonder that an enormous amount of hype surrounds these products. Millions of dollars are spent each year on pills and capsules, salves and ointments, yet there is little scientific knowledge on the buyer's part of how they work or how effective they truly are.

Among the medical, scientific, and nutritional communities, there is still controversy over the role that these supplements may play in promoting good health. Many seemingly authoritative diet and nutrition books discuss vitamins and minerals as if everything were already known about them. In reality, most of the claims are based on fantasy, the fad of the moment, misinterpretation of scientific evidence, or just plain greed.

Vitamins, Vitamins, and More Vitamins

The truth is, vitamins are great for promoting good health, but they're best consumed in their natural form (that is, by eating vitamin-rich foods). Supplements have not been shown to have any significant role in fighting cancer, contrary to what many nutritional experts assume.

When I first began research on these issues over ten years ago, I and many other medical authorities advocated the use of vitamins A, C, and E in pill form. Unfortunately, the reality was different, as I'll explain.

※ ※ ※

The anti-cancer vitamin craze began with studies that showed that people who never developed cancer had higher than average levels of vitamins A, C, and E in their bodies. Similarly, those who went on to develop the disease were often lacking in these vitamins. So many experts mistakenly assumed that supplements could prevent cancer.

In the last few years, several of the vitamin supplementation researchers have reported their results. Unfortunately, and surprisingly, these studies have shown that these vitamin supplements do not have much of an effect on overall health. In fact, those studies looking at vitamin A have not only been negative, but also indicated that at the dosage that vitamin A was prescribed, there seemed to be an *increase in the incidence of lung cancer in the patients on vitamin supplementation!* Scientists have learned from studies such as these that in order for vitamins to provide a protective barrier against disease, they must be consumed in their natural form as part of food; taking a supplement does not have the same beneficial effect.

It's not the vitamins themselves, though. Scientists have come to the conclusion after these studies that foods rich in vitamins A, C, and E also must contain another substance that protects the body from cancer and heart disease. In other words, the protective factor is something traveling *along* with the known vitamins. Research seems to be saying that you're much better off eating a carrot than taking vitamin A pills.

As I've already mentioned, vitamins A, C, and E are found in abundance in fruits and vegetables. Vitamin C is found in citrus fruits; vitamin

A is found in green, orange, and yellow vegetables; and vitamin E is found in leafy green and yellow vegetables, fish, poultry, and noncitrus fruits.

Listed below are some specific foods you'll want to add to your grocery list.

TABLE 8A

LIST OF EFFECTIVE CANCER FIGHTERS

Foods Rich in Vitamin A

Apricots	Beet greens	Bok choy	Bran
Broccoli	Salad greens	Corn	Crabmeat
Kale	Oatmeal	Sweet potatoes	Spinach
Tomatoes	Peaches	Cantaloupe	Carrots
Turnip greens	Pumpkins	Watermelons	Squash
Mangoes	Papayas	Brussels sprouts	

Foods Rich in Vitamin C

Apricots	Artichokes	Asparagus	Bananas
Beets	Berries	Sprouts	Cabbage
Cantaloupes	Cauliflower	Collard greens	Grapefruit
Mangoes	Oranges	Papayas	Plantains
Spinach	Mustard greens	Strawberries	Tomatoes
Turnip greens	Turnips	Lemons	Sweet potatoes
Kiwi	Broccoli	Kale	Green peppers
Brussels sprouts			

Foods Rich in Vitamin E

Broccoli	Leafy greens	Green peas	Oatmeal
Wheat germ	Fish oils	Fish	Yellow veggies
Poultry	Corn	Fruits, noncitrus	

But before you throw those vitamin bottles away...I don't mean to mislead you into thinking that vitamin and mineral pills are completely useless. Although they haven't been rigorously shown to have any effect on fighting cancer, some vitamins in pill form may still be beneficial to your health. Vitamin E, for instance, may favorably affect risk of heart disease and stroke. On the other hand, if for some reason you are deficient in certain vitamins because they're missing from your diet, it's very important to take these supplements (for instance, strict vegetarians may need to take B12 and folate).

How much you ought to take, and even if you should take any, is still the subject of intense debate and, unfortunately, there is not room in this book to cover the topic adequately. In brief, there is some link between antioxidants, heart disease, and cancer, but medical science hasn't yet figured it out.

A word of warning: Certain vitamins in high doses (vitamin A, for example) can be extremely toxic. Other vitamins and minerals taken in mega-doses simply go to waste. For instance, any dose of vitamin C over 200 milligrams per day is flushed out through the urine. So those who advocate mega-doses of this vitamin are not promoting good health; rather, they're promoting sales of vitamin C (not to mention the diarrhea caused by taking too much of this vitamin).

"What about Recommended Daily Allowances?" you may be asking about now. Recommended Daily Allowances (RDAs), which are set by the government and its scientific bodies, state the minimum daily amount of a vitamin or mineral that is considered "adequate." The problem with these recommended doses is that they do not state the amount required for optimal health—just the quantity needed to prevent deficiency. In other words, if you consume the RDA of vitamin "X," you won't have to worry about getting an illness caused by a deficiency of "X"—but you won't necessarily be getting all the vitamin "X" that your body needs.

So what is the optimal dose of a vitamin? The truth is, no one knows for certain. There is still much debate within the medical community about using vitamins in pill form. What I've tried to do is present you with the most up-to-date information available. Keeping these facts in mind, I hope you'll decide for yourself if you want to add them to your diet. Personally, I use very few supplements.

Eicasopentanoic Acid Is a Lot Better Than It Sounds

Remember that cod liver oil your mother forced you to take when you were young? Eicasopentanoic Acid (EPA) is essentially the same thing. EPA was discovered when scientists found that Eskimos had a very low incidence of arteriosclerosis in spite of the surprising fact that their intake of fat was high. The reason: Eskimos were eating high quantities of fish, and the oil found in these fish had a protective quality that seems to come from EPA. Researchers have since learned that EPA has the ability to lower the level of cholesterol in the blood, make platelets more slippery, act as an anticoagulant, and benefit the body in other ways. Although these findings are promising, there are a few things you should consider before you rush out to stock up on EPA capsules.

Expense—A jar of 90 capsules will cost you around $12.

Dosage—To get the same amount of EPA that an Eskimo consumes in a day, you'd have to take about 50 capsules.

Side-effects—EPA is known to interfere with the blood's normal clotting mechanisms. It can cause bleeding if taken in doses over a gram and may be to blame for the Eskimos' high incidence of strokes.

If you choose to supplement your diet with EPA, do so in moderation. Tell your health-care provider what you're doing! Now, with the possibility of serious side effects, why would anyone want to take EPA capsules? Some people feel that the benefits outweigh the risks. Personally, I prefer to get my EPA naturally—by eating fish several times a week. One serving of salmon is worth many EPA pills, and it's so much more delicious!

Aspirin May Cure More Than a Headache

Aspirin is one of the greatest drugs ever discovered. Not only is it a wonderful pain reliever, but it can also reduce the risk for a variety of illnesses, including heart attacks, strokes, and certain types of cancer. Studies have shown that patients who took one low-dose aspirin every day dramatically reduced their heart attack rates. More recently, aspirin has been shown to decrease the incidence of cancer of the large intestine and the esophagus.

Does this mean that you should start taking aspirin on a daily basis? I think so. Most authorities currently suggest taking one to two baby aspirins per day, and I feel this is a great addition to the Evolutionary Diet. However, I must caution you not to overuse this helpful drug. Aspirin (a molecule known as acetyl-salicylate) inhibits the clotting process. This can be beneficial in preventing hardening of the arteries, but when taken in large quantities, aspirin can also cause bleeding. This is especially true for people who have ulcers or small tumors in the intestines. Aspirin may also accent normal bruising. Check with your doctor to be sure you don't have any potential risk factors.

Salicylates are found naturally in certain foods (especially in spices); however, these salicylates may not possess the same anti-clotting, anti-heart disease, or anti-cancer effects as aspirin. Aspirin is, as we have said, *acetyl*-salicylate. It is the acetyl part of aspirin that is the active part of the molecule. In foods, salicylates may not be in the acetyl form and therefore may not have any beneficial qualities.

Fruits, Vegetables, and Fiber

Fruits and vegetables are full of vitamins, are wonderful cancer fighters, and are also great sources of fiber. By following the plan outlined in this book, you will naturally be consuming the right amount of produce. When you cut down the amount of animal fat you consume, your intake of legumes, fruits, and vegetables will increase in proportion. This is one of many advantages basic to the Evolutionary Diet.

Fiber is another great cancer fighter. In addition to making you regular (and preventing hemorrhoids), fiber decreases your risk for cancer of the colon, heart disease, stroke, and atherosclerosis. Fiber is also a great weight reducer because it adds bulk to your diet without adding any calories.

Fiber's benefits stem from the fact that it's largely indigestible (that's why it doesn't have any calories). It's the supporting structure of vegetables, legumes, fruits, whole grains, nuts, and cereals. (Fiber is also found in lesser quantities in meat, fish, and poultry.) Fiber works to fight colon cancer by increasing the bulk of the stool. It sops up water and other substances and keeps the stool in a more liquid form. So any cancer promoting agents that might be in the intestines are diluted into harmless concentrations. Fiber lowers your cholesterol level in much the same way. In the intestines, fiber combines with cholesterol, bile acids, and other fatty acids and removes them from the body.

The positive effects of fiber have been documented time and time again. Studies conducted in Finland, Israel, and San Francisco have all produced the same results: Geographic areas with high-fiber diets have low rates of colon cancer. Similarly, low-fiber diets increase the risk for developing cancer of the large intestine. We estimate that primitive hunter-gatherers ate about 45 grams of fiber per day. Yet most Americans eat half that amount!

Foods high in fiber are abundant and easily obtained. Cereals, grains, vegetables, nuts, and fruits are not only high in fiber but are potent sources of beneficial substances including carotenoids (vitamin A-like substances). However, processed high-fiber foods sometimes also contain a lot of sugar, salt, and fat. One popular breakfast cereal, for instance, has about 300 milligrams of sodium per ounce. A well-known "100 percent natural" cereal contains 41 percent fat, while another granola-type cereal has 35 percent fat. So read labels carefully!

How will you know when you're eating enough fiber? Do you have to count the grams of fiber in your diet? No, you just have to look in the toilet bowl for the answer. If your stool is loose, and either breaks up in the bowl spontaneously, or during flushing, you are probably taking in enough fiber. (When you start eating a high-fiber diet, you may think that you have diarrhea, yet slightly loose stools are normal!) So don't shy away from looking in the toilet bowl. Anything that comes out of your body is a potential source of information about what's going on inside of you. Take advantage of this opportunity to learn more about yourself!

The Benefits of Exercise

Even though *The Evolutionary Diet and Cookbook* is primarily about food, I want to include a few words about the benefits of exercise. In addition to making you look good, exercise also makes you feel great. Even better, countless studies show that exercise benefits your health by:

- lowering blood cholesterol;
- increasing vitality;
- burning calories for weight loss; and
- reducing the risk of heart disease.

There are all sorts of exercise gurus who will tell you about the physiologic changes that occur when you exercise, but how much, how often, and how to exercise are outside the scope of this book. What I will urge you to do, though, is to take a daily brisk walk for at least 20 minutes, enough to make you perspire.

Tobacco Is Harmful

This is another topic that, like exercise, needs only a few words. I can think of two choice ones: **DON'T SMOKE!**

※ ※ ※ ※ ※ ※

Chapter Nine

Shopping Like a Cro-Magnon and Reading Labels

"W hat should I make for dinner?" It's a question that our primitive ancestors never had to ask—simply because they didn't have much choice in the matter. Their dinner consisted of what their environment provided them with—what they had found or caught that day. We, on the other hand, are constantly bombarded with eating choices. Not only do we get to decide what restaurant we patronize, we're faced with a wide array of dishes once we get there.

At the grocery store, making choices is even harder because there's even more to choose from. Here we see tens of thousands of different foods, some of which are healthy, but most of which are either processed in some way or would never appear on earth naturally.

So how do you think like a Cro-Magnon in the supermarket? The first step is to ask yourself what you would be eating if you could only hunt (wild game, crustacea, birds, or fish) or gather things (fruits, vegetables, and seeds) as our early ancestors did. It's actually a lot easier than you might think.

Perimeter Shopping

Learning to shop like a Cro-Magnon is simply a lesson in geography. Why? Because grocery stores are organized in the same way as our society. Think about where you live. If you live in a city, you're at the center of business, government, and manufacturing. If you've settled in the country, you live outside the center; you're on the outskirts. Now think about the kind of food that comes from these two distinct places. From the country, we get fresh fruits and vegetables and meat. In the city, this food is processed and packaged.

The grocery store is laid out in the same way. In the center, you find "city food," which generally has been altered in some form. Along the outskirts of the market, you shop for produce and meats. As you've probably already guessed, your best strategy is to shop the perimeter of the store. Here is where you will find the majority of healthy foods that should make up your diet. Personally, I rarely go up and down the aisles unless I need oil, condiments, or paper towels.

The only items on the perimeter that you might be wary of are those that contain the products of domesticated animals—cheese, cream, milk, and eggs, for example.

If you venture into the center of the market, BEWARE of processed foods. As you already know, Cro-Magnons did not eat processed foods simply because these items were not available back then. Although we do have them around in great quantities, we should follow our early ancestors' lead and avoid most of these foods entirely. In general, they are loaded with salt and fat.

Nutritionists tend to say that food additives are dangerous. The Evolutionary Diet naturally avoids additives and processed foods (with a few exceptions).

On Reading Labels

The format of the current nutritional information labels seems to be more of a lesson in politics and influence than an informational and educational tool. For your amazement, amusement and, most of all, for your education, here are a few samples of labels.

Let's use as our first example the label on so-called 2% milk. Here we will be able to see the basic elements of the "Nutrition Facts."

FIGURE 9A

2% MILK PRODUCT NUTRITIONAL LABEL

Nutrition Facts

Serving Size 1cup (240mL)
Servings Per Container About 2

Amount Per Serving

Calories 140	Calories from Fat 45
	% Daily Value*

Total Fat 5g	**8%**
Saturated Fat 3.5g	**18%**
Cholesterol 30mg	**10%**
Sodium 130mg	**5%**
Total Carbohydrate 13g	**4%**
Dietary Fiber 0g	**0%**
Sugars 13g	
Protein 10g	**20%**

Vitamin A 10%	• Vitamin C 4%	•	Calcium 30%
Iron 0%	•		Vitamin D 25%

*Percent Daily Values are based on a 2,000 calorie diet. Your daily values may be higher or lower depending on your caloric needs:

	Calories:	2,000	2,500
Total Fat	Less than	65g	80g
Sat. Fat	Less than	20g	25g
Cholesterol	Less than	300mg	300mg
Sodium	Less than	2,400mg	2,400mg
Total Carbohydrates		300g	375g
Dietary Fiber		25g	30g
Protein		50g	65g

First, notice that the name of the product is not on the nutritional label (other than the word *milk* at the bottom, which doesn't help to tell us if this is skim milk, 1% milk, 2% milk, or whole milk). The front of the carton says 2%. But note that the nutritional "fact chart" on the back has no such number printed. "What is 2% milk, and how do I find out? All these other numbers and percentages are confusing!" And who wouldn't be confused? A little later, I'll show you how to find out what the *real* percent of 2% milk is.

Reading nutritional labels, for many people, is probably as interesting as the fine print on a contract. Food manufacturers make use of this apathy by printing something on the face of the product (here, 2% milk) and then giving the important nutritional information hidden on the back label. It's hidden, because if the calculation of percentage of calories as fat was made for us, we would see how nutritionally dangerous some products are. Fortunately, enough information is provided so that we can calculate that percentage of calories from fat we so vitally need to know.

How to Calculate the Percentage of Calories from Fat

Most people look at a nutritional label to see how many calories per serving something contains. However, unless you are conducting food research, the only number of real importance is the one that's usually NOT listed on the label: the percentage of the total calories that come from fat. Luckily, we are given information on the package of most foods that makes it easy to calculate this percentage.

First, look at portion size. Here, it's one cup (240 ml.).

The next line is the most important. It will enable us to calculate the percentage of the total calories from fat very easily. Here, each serving of milk has 130 calories, and 45 of these calories are from fat. What percentage is fat? Easy: 45 divided by 130 = 0.346 = 34.6%! Hey, I thought that this was 2% milk. What happened? My calculation shows almost 35% fat in milk—and I have new batteries in my calculator. What does this mean?

It's quite simple: The milk industry wants you to pay more attention to the 2% figure. In this way you'll think that you're getting a low-fat product. The calculation is true and valid; you are not being lied to, but it is brazenly misleading. Here's how the 2% calculation is done: If percentage of fat is calculated as percent of total *weight*, not percent of total *calories*, the number calculated is much smaller. Yet, it is the percent of *calories* from fat that is the biologically relevant number. In our 2% milk example, a serving is close to 240 cc's. The label informs us that there are 5 grams of fat per serving. So divide the 5 grams by the 240 grams, and we get 2% of weight as fat. But this number is of no importance.

Look at it this way: If I took one gram of oil and put it into 100 grams of water, then by *weight*, this mixture would be 1% fat. But, because water doesn't have any calories, 100% of the calories would be in the form of fat. The 2% milk is a variant of this trick. It is really almost 35% calories from fat.

Let's look at the label further.

The *Daily Value* is supposed to be another improvement in nutritional labeling. Personally, I think that it's confusing and misleading to the unwary. As you saw, we read the 2% value on the milk carton, yet calculated 34.6% as the actual nutritional fat percentage. But here, look in the "daily value" section—it says fat is 8%! So now we have three numbers to contend with, and each one of those numbers claims to be accurately and authoritatively describing the fat content of this milk. How can this be? Well, it all depends on your point of view. If we want to measure by weight, we get 2%. If we measure by calories (the metabolically correct way), we get 34.6% and, as we shall see, when we calculate it as a percentage of what is called "Daily Value," we will get 8%.

The Daily Value is based on the estimated or ideal number of calories that the average person eats per day. This has been set, for purposes of labeling, at a calorie intake of 2,000 or 2,500 calories per day for women and men. The amount of fat allowed is calculated in the following way: If the calorie intake is supposed to be 2,000 calories, and the USDA recommendations are for no more than 30% of the calories from fat, then (30% of 2,000) 600 calories can come from fat. Because a gram of fat contains 9 calories, dividing the 600 by 9 will give us the number of grams of fat "permitted" per day. This is 66.6 grams, but here it is rounded off to 65. (See it at the bottom of the label?) Under these rules, we can eat up to 65 grams of fat per day.

So how does this get us to the 8 percent? Here's how: There are 5 grams of fat in one serving of this milk. Therefore, what percentage is 5 grams? If total fat permitted per day is 65 grams (the Daily Value), then $5/65 \times 100 = 7.692$ percent, but rounded up to 8 percent. Of course you must be eating 2,000 calories per day and must be at a total of 30 percent of calories as fat. Using these numbers forces you to calculate every calorie and every gram of fat to make sure that it all adds up. I recommend that you pay attention to the biologically and physiologically most important percentage, and that is the percentage of total calories from fat *in that particular food item*. Forget about calculating every calorie for the whole day; you'll get a headache, if not bored or confused.

Thirty percent of calories per day from fat is probably too high, and a 2,000-calorie-a-day diet may be okay for a woman who is "x" pounds and "x" inches tall. But what happens if you are "y" pounds and "y" inches tall? The same numbers will not apply.

Our government, through its scientific bodies, has recommended no more than 30 percent of calories from fat in the American diet. Cro-Magnon hunter-gatherers probably ate less than a 25-percent-fat diet. Tasty dishes can be prepared at about 25 percent fat without a feeling of deprivation. I suggest you gradually reduce your fat. But don't do this "cold turkey." With a little practice, you can "eyeball" the figures and won't actually have to sit down with paper and pencil or a calculator. But you'll know when you're cheating—and that's every time you have dairy (other than nonfat) or most domestic red meat.

Getting back to the label—look at the Daily Value of vitamins. Here is another percentage that is confusing and not helpful. If a serving contains 10 percent of my Daily Value of vitamin A, what does that mean? Ten percent of what? How much vitamin A am I getting? If it's the daily value, I am not told what the total amount of vitamin A per day "should" be. (Then, there is the additional issue of what the right dose of vitamin A is. This question, along with minimum daily requirements, has been discussed in chapter eight.)

In my opinion, Daily Value is not a helpful addition to the label.

Let's move on from the ridiculous to the sublime and look at Figure 9B. It's the label of a spray product that you can use for greasing pans. Let's see how much information there is here.

FIGURE 9B

VEGETABLE OIL SPRAY—PRODUCT NUTRITIONAL LABEL

Nutrition Facts

Serving Size About
$1/3$ Second Spray (.266g)
Servings Per Container About 453

Amount Per Serving	
Calories 0	Calories from Fat 0
	% Daily Value*
Total Fat 0g	0%
Saturated Fat 0g	0%
Cholesterol 0mg	0%
Sodium 0mg	0%
Total Carbohydrate 0g	0%
Protein 0g	0%

Not a significant source of dietary fiber, sugars, vitamin A, vitamin C, calcium and iron.

*Percent Daily Values are based on a 2,000 calorie diet.

Note that this product has zero calories and therefore zero calories from fat. Hey, hold on. Wait just a minute! Isn't the main ingredient of this spray canola oil? See the asterisk? It says that using this product "adds a trivial amount of oil." The statement may be true, but the labeling is misleading. I called up the company that makes this product, and they admitted to me that close to 100 percent of the spray that sticks to the pan is in the form of oil (that's fat). So how can the label state "zero percent"? The secret is in the serving size.

The serving size has been set or proclaimed to be one-third of a second spray, in which .266 grams of fat are released. This means that we have .266 grams x 9 calories/gram = 2.4 calories in each third-of-a-second spray. Of course 2.4 calories is not much—and I am not grousing over a mere 2-plus calories. But the fat content is registered as zero percent! What gives? Well, it turns out that if the *amount* (in weight) of the substance in a serving is less than one-half a gram (here .266 of a gram), then federal regulations allow the resulting number to be rounded off to zero! In reality, consider how you spray a pan if you use this product. A third of a second spray is too little to coat a pan. Many users will spray at least three times this amount, for about one second. In the real world, the use per serving will be about .8 of a gram, and this would merit a notation that 100 percent of calories are from fat.

I agree that the total amount of fat is low. My concern is that the average consumer looking at the Nutritional Value label will think that there is no fat in the spray. This confusion exists only because of "rounding down." Any serving less than half a gram is equal to zero. Go figure!

❖ ❖ ❖

Here's another food label. It's one that you've seen many times. It's so common that I'll just print it here:

Leanest Ground Beef
15 Percent Fat

Well, what do you think about this label? After studying the two previous examples, you're pretty skeptical, aren't you? Me, too. We both know that this is not really 15 percent calories from fat. It's 15 percent by weight of the product. But many grams of the meat do not have any caloric value (water, fiber, sinew) and are not digestible. Therefore, it is the same type of problem as the "2%" milk label.

Cuts of domesticated beef with 15 percent fat by *weight* can be found. These include lean rib eye, braised lean bottom round, round tip, and so on. But let's calculate what this number really means in terms of percentage of calories from fat. The average piece of 100 grams (3.5 oz) of a 15-percent-fat meat has about 250 calories. Therefore, it has 15 grams of fat (15 percent of 100). If a gram of fat = 9 calories, there will be a total of 135 calories from fat. Then, 135 calories from fat are divided by the 250 total calories, and we get an amazing 54 percent of calories from fat. So much for lean! And 15 percent is the leanest domesticated meat you can regularly get in a supermarket.

So my advice is: It's okay to splurge once in a while. But remember that you're eating over 50 percent fat calories when you eat a lean hamburger. A whole steak may be even higher in fat. If you want red meat, it's better to get wild game, venison, ostrich, and the like. Keep in mind that meticulous de-fatting of meat by aggressive trimming and then grilling or broiling will decrease fat content markedly.

The take-home lesson about labels is that we can use them to calculate the percentage of total calories that are from fat. The rest of the information is relatively useless unless you record the amount of everything you eat.

❊ ❊ ❊

Not all food labeling is as simple as the examples cited above. There are two other terms you should be aware of. The first is a label that says something such as "98 percent fat free." Of course, by now you're probably as cynical as I am about these labels and know that although the statement is true, it does not give us any information that is practical. Ninety-eight percent fat free is the other side of the two percent milk story. Providers of milk could just as easily proclaim two percent milk as being 98 percent fat free!

Finally, the other commonly seen label is: "No cholesterol." This means what it says. There is no cholesterol in the product. This notation is usually found on oils. However, it is misleading, too. The assumption on the part of the consumer is that the oils that do not have such wording on the label are filled with cholesterol. This is another trick. No food made from plant products has cholesterol. Cholesterol is ONLY found in animal products. You should, of course, recognize that while oils do not have any cholesterol, they do contain fat. The no-cholesterol label is the equivalent of putting the label "No Fat" on a package of cigarettes. It's true, but not really helpful or applicable.

There are some other variations on these themes of food labels. However, these are decreasing in number as manufacturers are forced to give us more data.

My advice: Read carefully, calculate, or "eyeball" the percentage of fat calories. Then let your good sense and conscience be your guide.

Final Shopping Notes

The small amount of searching it may take to find certain items (such as animal protein) will reward you in the end by providing you with a lifetime free of the diseases most people face in old age. Besides, finding Evolutionary foods in the supermarket is getting easier every day. Grocery stores are beginning to offer a wider selection of specialty items, and gourmet markets are carrying an increasingly diverse choice of fowl, meat, vegetables, and fruit, some of which are perfect for our food requirements.

Remember, you don't have to go to the supermarket, calculator in hand, and figure out the percentage of fat for each item in your cart. Shop the perimeter of the store (remembering to avoid the dairy section), and you won't have to. But if you decide to venture into the interior of the supermarket, from time to time you should figure out the fat contents of a few of these foods. After a while, with a little experience you'll get a sense of what's acceptable and what's best left on the shelf.

❈ ❈ ❈ ❈ ❈ ❈

Chapter Ten
(for Women)

From a Woman's Point of View

I asked my wife, Kathye, to write this chapter to give a woman's perspective on how to make the Evolutionary Diet a part of your life.

※ ※ ※

Author's Note:

This chapter is really about and for our female readers. Although our male readers are welcome to read it, please be aware that you may not identify with the some of the comments in the chapter or find them appropriate for you.

※ ※ ※

How We Measure Up to Our Cro-Magnon Counterparts

Cro-Magnon women certainly didn't spend the time, energy, and money that we modern women do to make ourselves beautiful. They lived without the aid of cosmetics, designer clothes, and hair stylists. Yet, my guess is that they had the good complexions, shiny hair, and trim bodies we seek. Imagine accomplishing all that naturally!

True, our Cro-Magnon sisters didn't have to deal with modern-day beauty-wreckers such as desk jobs with long hours and pizza delivery services. But we have the same genes (that's DNA, not Levis). Cro-Magnon women underwent the same hormonal fluctuations that sometimes encourage changes in our complexions and our weight. They went through puberty, pregnancy, and regular (or irregular) menstrual periods. They nursed their babies and may have lived long enough to experience menopause.

But if we spent a fraction of the time that it takes making ourselves artificially beautiful with makeup, clothes, and new hair colors, and invested it in our health, we would find ourselves looking more beautiful naturally.

Now, don't get me wrong. I enjoy having my hair done and shopping for new clothes as much as most women do. But I find that when I am at my healthiest, I am also at my most beautiful. My hair is shiny, my complexion is clear, my body is firm, my energy level is higher, and I feel better about myself. How to get there without too much pain, hunger, and suffering is the real issue, and that is exactly what this chapter is all about.

The Realities of Dieting

My husband, Ron, has touched on some of the problems with most diets (for instance, the more bizarre or difficult the diet, the less likely we are to stay on it). As women, many of us try these diets in those very real moments of truth, such as when we realize that we have put on a few pounds over the winter and we have a bathing suit to get into the next month. We often find ourselves dieting to get into a certain dress to wear to a certain event. And proudly, after eating nothing but grapefruit and papaya for weeks, we can get into that dress or even that swimsuit. Then, of course, we stop the diet and slowly but surely (or sometimes not so slowly), ounce by ounce, and then pound by pound, we go right back to where we started.

Since I began work on this chapter, I've been talking to a lot of women about calories and weight. One of the topics that comes up frequently is how we, as intelligent, sophisticated women, are capable of deceiving ourselves. So I've compiled a list of the top ten ways we like to fool ourselves when it comes to dieting and calories:

1. There are no calories in broken cookies.
2. I'm overweight right now because I'm getting my period. (It's just water weight.)
3. Now that I've lost five pounds, I can reward myself with a hamburger and a shake.
4. If I have several dress sizes in my closet, I will always be well dressed.
5. Eating in the car while driving doesn't count.
6. It's okay to eat as much as I want as long as it's nonfat.
7. When I eat at a restaurant, it's fine to ignore everything I ever learned about healthy eating.
8. As soon as I get back into a size "x," I can stop dieting.
9. There are no calories in food or liquor when you're on vacation.
10. A Diet Coke will nullify the calories in a piece of chocolate cake.

And then there's the battle with the scales. It seems that we always try to weigh ourselves when there's the slightest chance we may be a pound or two thinner. Some examples:

1. Right after going to the bathroom
2. Before eating or drinking anything
3. Always after exercising
4. After our periods, never before
5. After getting a haircut, clipping our nails, and shaving our legs
6. Always when we're naked

Obviously I mean these lists to be funny, but quite frankly, it makes me realize that I and many other women have been approaching this weight and physical beauty thing all wrong. My husband, Ron, believes we should follow the Evolutionary plan outlined in this book to avoid cancer and heart disease, and I think he's right. But until I knew him, I didn't realize that following his simple guidelines with the addition of a little exercise (even walking or shopping), would drastically change my body and the way I looked. And it happened accidentally.

Over the course of a few months of being on the Evolutionary Diet, I watched my energy level increase dramatically. Before that time, I often came home exhausted after a ten-hour day at the office. All I wanted was some sugar to give me energy. Sugar in the form of ice cream or a glass of wine were my favorites; of course, the energy lasted only about as long as the ice cream. I was too exhausted to even take a walk.

But once I began eating correctly and my energy level increased, I became interested in integrating a bit of physical activity into my life. A walk after dinner and a few ballet exercises on weekends became natural and fun. My clothes started getting looser, and my friends began to notice.

When Ron first told me about his way of eating to be healthy, I thought it sounded reasonable, but the thought of *never* eating ice cream again defied my reality. Yet, after two to three weeks of following the Evolutionary Diet, I stopped craving some of the foods I was used to, mostly those filled with fat and sugar. After that, no one could have talked me into going back to my old, unhealthy habits. I just kept getting healthier. And soon I could even look at my naked body without closing one or both eyes.

When I think about it in retrospect, I must admit that, back then, the changes in my looks and my energy were most important to me. Now I realize that the improvement in my health has had a much more profound effect. For several generations, many of my family members have died young of cancer, heart disease, and complications from diabetes, and I had put myself on the same path. More important, I had been poisoning my body and putting myself at risk for dying young; I was following in the family tradition quite needlessly.

How to Get Started on Your Health and Beauty Plan

Based on my own experiences, I've come up with a list of eight tips to help you uncover the healthy and beautiful woman that lies within you.

1. FOLLOW DR. CITRON'S EVOLUTIONARY DIET PLAN.

   I believe you'll be pleasantly surprised by how easy this plan is to follow. One of the reasons it's so effective is that it's reasonable and you can adhere to it anywhere—no buying special diet foods, no inconveniencing your hostess or waiter.

   Remember, you may have cravings for certain foods (especially those filled with fat and sugar) for a few weeks. Expect it, but know it will pass. If you feel a little hungry, have a piece of fruit or a green salad with vinegar or a little skinless chicken or fish to get you through that initial stage. Also, remember that it's okay to be a little hungry; you'll know your body is burning up those fat calories and starting to get healthy.

2. A SAMPLE WEEK—MENUS TO GET YOU STARTED.

   Following the guidelines outlined in the Evolutionary Diet is enough to put you on the path to good health. But for those of you who need to structure your life-change program, I've included seven days of lunches, dinners, and suggested snacks. Recipes for these menus can be found in the second half of this book. These menus are made up of recipes that are particularly low in fat and calories. The menus also provide a perfect "getting back on track" week after you've been vacationing and eating at restaurants that sneak fat into their food even when you're trying to avoid it. If you're like me, a week of eating these delicious foods will convince you that eating to create a healthy, beautiful you is much less difficult than you thought it would be.

   Unless otherwise noted, all recipes can be found in the recipe section of the book.

❈ ❈ ❈

DAY ONE

Lunch

KATHYE'S FAVORITE SALAD

We might as well start out righteous by having a "diet" salad. Actually, you'll find that this salad is very filling; I usually eat it for lunch two or three times a week. It's so simple that it isn't in the cookbook section. Here's what I do:

Chop a shallot or a clove of garlic and place in a BIG bowl with 1 Tbsp. balsamic vinegar, 1 Tbsp. wine vinegar, a pinch of salt, pepper, and sugar. Sometimes I add ½ tsp Dijon mustard or 1 Tbsp. HoMade (brand name) Chili Sauce. Mix well. Now cut up your favorite lettuce or romaine. Toss it with any or all of the following: 2 green onions, chopped; 1 hard-boiled egg (the white only because the yolk is high in fat), chopped; 1 stalk celery, chopped; ½ tomato, chopped; ¼ cup non-fat cottage cheese (with extra salt and pepper); some green beans, broccoli, or cauliflower, and so on. In other words, put in any vegetable you like. Toss and enjoy. The textures are wonderful, it takes forever to eat and, best of all, it has almost no calories (less than 100) and NO fat.

Dinner

GRILLED SWORDFISH WITH TOMATO SAUCE (pg. 263)
STEAMED RICE
BANANA PARFAIT (pg. 311)

Snack

(Anytime during the day when those hunger pangs start getting to you)

A SMOOTHIE (pg. 308)

DAY TWO

Lunch

SALMON TARTARE (pg. 172)

Dinner

BBQ ROAST TURKEY SANDWICHES

Make these fabulous sandwiches, and your family will never believe you're dieting! Roast your own turkey breast, if possible (pg. 272). Make the Creamy Slaw (pg. 200) and the Lowfat Barbeque Sauce (pg. 315). Heat the sauce, and spread generously on both sides of hamburger buns. Heap with turkey and add more sauce if you like a messy barbeque. Top the turkey with some of that good slaw. (I like my barbeque sauce a little spicier than the recipe, so I add a few shakes of cayenne pepper while heating the sauce.)

VANILLA PEACHES (pg. 308)

Snack

A SLICE OF WATERMELON AND/OR AN ORANGE

DAY THREE

Lunch

LARB (pg. 175)
(Walk on the wild side, if you've
never tried it. It's like popcorn...you'll want more.)

Dinner

"TWO CUP" MUSHROOM BARLEY SOUP (pg. 186)
RATATOUILLE (pg. 221)
SLICED PINEAPPLE

Snack

1/4 CUP NONFAT COTTAGE CHEESE AND/OR AN APPLE

DAY FOUR

Lunch

KATHYE'S FAVORITE HAMBURGER

(This is a little like the salad—not worthy of a recipe, but really good.)

Take a hamburger bun (I heat mine in the microwave) and spread with your favorite condiments: mustard, catsup, pickle relish (but no mayo). Top with traditional fillings such as tomatoes, red onions, lettuce, and pickles. Then in place of the beef patty, use $1/4$ cup nonfat cottage cheese.)

Dinner

CREAMED CORN SOUP (pg. 184)
STEAMED FISH (pg. 254)

Snack

SALSA WITH RAW VEGGIES (pg. 159)

Day Five

Lunch

OPEN-FACED CRAB SANDWICHES (pg. 246)

Dinner

CORN-STUFFED CHILIES (pg. 216)
RAYMOND'S GARLIC CHICKEN (pg. 277)

Snack

A SMOOTHIE (pg. 308)

DAY SIX

Lunch

PUMPKIN SOUP (pg. 185)
SALAD GREENS WITH LEMON JUICE

Dinner

CAJUN DIRTY RICE WITH SHRIMP (pg. 249)
SALAD OF GRAPEFRUIT, ORANGE, FENNEL (pg. 202)

Snack

SOFT TACO
(Here I go again, a recipe with no recipe.) This is a 100-calorie snack.
Have two tacos and call it lunch. Take a corn tortilla and spread with 2
Tbsp. nonfat cream cheese. Heat for 45 seconds in the microwave. Top
with tomatoes, red onions, lettuce, and Tabasco sauce.

DAY SEVEN

Lunch

STEAMED ARTICHOKE STUFFED WITH
SHRIMP OR CRAB (pg. 208)

Dinner
(good when you have company)

MOC-GUACAMOLE WITH CELERY STICKS (pg. 158)
LOBSTER AND ARTICHOKE SALAD (pg. 214)
BBQ SWORDFISH (pg. 262)
VEGETABLE COUSCOUS (pg. 228)
APPLE-PEAR WITH KIWI SAUCE (pg. 309)

Snack
(You probably won't be hungry, but if you are, a piece of fruit
or even some carrot sticks will do before your evening feast.)

P.S. NEVER GO TO THE MARKET WHEN
YOU'RE HUNGRY!

3. REWARD YOURSELF FOR YOUR EFFORTS IN PURSUIT OF GOOD HEALTH.

Probably the most important thing to remember as you begin eating for good health is that you're *not on a diet*; a diet is short-term—what you go through to fit into a swimsuit. The Evolutionary Diet is for life. It's a dramatic change in the way you view the foods you're putting into your body, and it will have a major impact on your life.

Embarking on any change can be tough, so reward yourself for your early successes. Start with a glamorous magazine, a facial, or a new pair of shoes after the first week. Make a list of rewards to treat yourself with on a regular basis and buy yourself a new bathing suit after three months. My guess is that long before the end of three months, your newly healthy beautiful body will be reward in itself.

4. WHEN EATING OUT, EAT HALF AS MUCH AS YOU'RE SERVED.

This is not a firm rule, but it's an easy guideline to follow when you're in a position where it's difficult to control the fat content in your food. My friend Jan showed me just how effective this simple tip can be. She had been a stewardess for many years, and keeping her weight down was important to her. She had always been thin and fit, but one day she broke her hip. Not able to exercise, she put on weight, more than she'd ever imagined. After the reality of her weight problem set in, Jan began eating half of whatever she was served—whether she was in a restaurant or a dinner guest in someone's home. Of course, she didn't know about the Evolutionary Diet then, but her approach worked well. By making this subtle change, she lost her excess weight nearly effortlessly.

5. BE AWARE OF PORTION SIZES.

Even though *counting calories* is not part of the Evolutionary Diet, *being aware of calories* is important. The reality is, the actual portions most of us eat (at home or in restaurants) are much larger than portions listed in most nutritional texts and on labels. For example, in most texts, serving portions for meats and fish are typically three ounces. For chicken, this would be about half a breast. That's right. So when you're enjoying a family barbeque and eating a barbequed chicken breast (skin removed, of course), just remember, you're eating two servings, not one. (This is where the "Eat half as much as you're served" tip comes in handy.)

When you begin making recipes from this book, take note of the portion sizes. If a recipe says it serves six, but at your table it only serves four, try recalculating the calories so you know just how many you really are consuming. Do the same thing with canned, frozen, and packaged foods from the market. From past experience, I've learned just how eye-opening this can be. For years I've tended to eat nonfat cottage cheese and salad greens with vinegar for lunch a couple of times a week (it's just something I've found that I like that is also quick and easy). But I'd never really measured the amount of cottage cheese I was eating. One day, I spooned some on a plate, figuring it was about a quarter of a cup (40 calories) and thinking I was being exceptionally "good." Just before I lifted my fork, I decided to see whether my perception and reality were the same. I was off by 100 percent. That nonfat cottage cheese portion was twice the amount I had assumed it was. (Of course, when you're eating nonfat cottage cheese, you don't really have to worry.) The point is that it's a good idea to measure the amount of food you're eating once in a while to reality-test—especially when you're eating foods that aren't low in fat. It's not that it's bad to eat more than "a portion" now and then; it's just good to be aware that you're doing it.

6.   EXERCISE WHILE YOU WATCH THE NEWS.

Instead of just sitting there on the sofa, get on that exercise bike, or do some yoga or sit-ups. Exercise has been proven to be beneficial to our health, particularly for maintaining healthy hearts. From my standpoint, the three best things about exercise are:

a) It makes me feel better. When I say this, I don't just mean it improves my self-esteem. Exercise actually changes my mood and helps me face my other daily challenges.

b) It raises my metabolism. Since Ron and I love to cook and (of course) eat, having a higher metabolism allows me to do what I love without paying the price of consuming fewer calories.

c) It's a lot more fun being firm than flabby!

You're probably saying to yourself, "Okay, okay, I know all that. Now back to reality." The truth is, in spite of its benefits, it's tough to exercise. These are some of my best excuses:

❋ **Excuse #1: Exercise is too time-consuming**. Even if you're a fast runner, exercise takes valuable time out of your day. I used to think of exercise as something that I'd treat myself to once I'd finished a project. But often the project wouldn't get done, or by the time I completed it, I was way too tired to exercise. It took me a while to realize how backward my thinking was. Now I exercise faithfully *before* I complete my projects. This gives me the extra energy I need to work, and it actually adds to my time—I no longer need to take naps. When I put my physical and emotional health first, I am more productive in my work and enjoy it more.

Of course there are times when exercise is unrealistic or I'm too busy. That's when I exercise while watching the news. Sometimes I stand in the kitchen waiting for the water to boil and do arm flexes. It sounds silly, but for me, any exercise is better than no exercise.

❋ **Excuse #2: Exercise is boring**. I'm a terrible tennis player, and repetitive exercises are boring to me. You, no doubt, have your own list of exercises that you're not particularly fond of. Of course, the answer is finding an exercise you enjoy. It doesn't really matter what you do as long as you do *something*. Ron and I go through funny phases like rollerblading or throwing horseshoes. We both have fun walking and have tied this activity to our evenings out. When we dine out, we often park two miles away from the restaurant and walk there and back. All over the world I've been seen wearing a fancy dress with tennis shoes. I stop outside the restaurant and put on my heels. No one is the wiser, except for me!

Finding a partner to work out with is another great tip. You'll find that exercise is more fun, and you'll encourage each other. As

I've already mentioned, Ron and I do much of our exercising together.

※ **Excuse #3: I can't get started.** The absolute worst part of exercising is getting started. I once drove to a gym, parked, sat in the car for ten minutes, and drove home. And there are times that are even more challenging, such as puberty, being married, being not married, being pregnant, just after being pregnant, menopause, when we're stressed out by family, or concerned about the job we have or don't have. Our emotional good health has an enormous impact on our physical good health and vice versa. After all, we may think we're having a "bad hair day" when in fact we look just fine; it's just that we feel lousy.

It's so much harder to improve our physical health when we're not feeling good about ourselves. This frustrating cycle is, of course, that it sometimes takes improving our physical health for us to become healthier emotionally. Sometimes we just forget how wonderful we truly are. Once we remember, everything becomes easier.

7. REMEMBER WHO YOU ARE.

    Have you ever noticed how beautiful a woman looks when she's in love or pregnant? Our mood affects our appearance, and when we're feeling happy, we actually look better. You can keep that beautiful glow if you work to be content with who you are. By feeling good about yourself, you'll find it easy to begin the Evolutionary Diet plan. You'll know you deserve the best, with good health and good looks. Below are some motivational tools to help you remember just how wonderful you are.

    a) **Affirm the positive**. For many years I ran a successful business that (among other things) dealt with women's issues in the labor market. On numerous occasions, I spoke to women's organizations and at conferences about techniques for getting a raise or landing the perfect job. In all my speeches, I emphasized the tremendous impact that personal affirmations can have in helping women get what we want. I encouraged participants to repeat positive personal statements out loud, to write them down and put them on their bathroom mirrors, and to tape-record them and play the recordings while they were in their cars. I know this advice worked, because time and time again, people wrote to me or told me in person that they had gotten the job, the raise, or whatever it was they had been seeking.

The irony was, I had seen the results for others, *but I had never taken my own advice!* Then came my own awakening. It happened on the day I mentioned previously, the day when I sat in my car in a gym parking lot, depressed and unable to move. After I had started the car and headed home, I decided I deserved to be depressed and to feel sorry for myself. Then it hit me: I was punishing myself, making myself miserable, and would probably pass this state on to those I loved. The fact that I knew that the thoughts and feelings I was having were absurd didn't help. What did help was *personal affirmation.*

I said to myself, "Kathye Citron, now it's your turn to practice what you preach." I looked at my reflection in the mirror (feeling more than a little silly) and started by saying, "I am wonderful, I am intelligent, I am pretty, I am sexy, I am successful, my body is good and getting better." All of a sudden as I repeated these things, I was smiling, I felt wonderful, and I was myself again. But there was one difference: I had learned an important lesson and had grown a little from it. I had used personal affirmations for myself, and they had worked. And I'm still using them.

b) **Use personal affirmations.** To start using personal affirmation in your own life, first make a list of the things about you that make you wonderful. Start with who you are. For example: "I am wonderful, I love myself, I am worthy, I am kind, I am a good person, I am a good friend, I am considerate, I am a good partner, I am a good mother, I am smart, I am resourceful." These are just a few ideas. After you come up with your own affirmations, ask your family and friends for other suggestions.

Tell them you're working on an exercise and need their input on your best attributes. You might be surprised. They may have some ideas for your list that you haven't even thought of. (Remember to always state your affirmations in the present tense. If you say, "I will get a great job" or something similar, then your goal will always remain in the future, just out of your reach.)

For the moment, write your first five affirmations here:

1. _____

2. _____

3. _____

4. _____

5. _____

Next, make a list of the things that you find beautiful about yourself. For example: "I have great ankles, I have beautiful hair, I have a beautiful smile, I have nice ears, I am beautiful inside and out." Once again, get some input. Then list five of them here to use as affirmations:

1. _____

2. _____

3. _____

4. _____

5. _____

Finally, make a list of where you are and where you're headed. For example: "I am getting healthy, I am getting thinner, I am fit and getting fitter, I am enjoying healthy eating." I've included the first affirmation for you. Write your own below it.

1. <u>I deserve to be healthy and beautiful.</u>

2. _____

3. _____

4. _____

5. _____

Now, congratulate yourself.

You have just taken the first step toward achieving health and beauty. Now, keep going. Keep smiling and repeating these affirmations until you feel comfortable. Write them down and put them on your refrigerator, and every time you're in your kitchen, repeat them. Write them down again and tape them to your bathroom mirror. Every morning when you get up and every night before you go to bed, repeat them, smiling.

By feeling good about yourself, you'll find it easy to begin the Evolutionary Diet plan. You'll know you deserve the best—good health, good looks, and a positive state of mind.

8. YOU HAVE THE POWER TO BE YOUR BEST. Remember the story of the rabbit and the hare, and give yourself the gift of time in order to be your best. Quick diets just don't work. When you start one of them, you feel desperate and out of control. However, when you embark on Dr. Citron's plan and acknowledge that real, substantial, and lasting change takes time, you feel powerful. Beginning a beautification program that lasts for life is like planting a garden. You'll see small changes that develop along the way. In three months, you'll really see a difference in the way you look and feel. Your energy level will be higher, and your clothes will fit better. Little by little, your body will have become its best. Now, what could be better than that? Not even a hot fudge sundae!

Chapter Eleven

Curing Disease

B y now, you should be seeing the world much as our Cro-Magnon ancestors viewed it. You're eating food provided by your natural environment, you're consuming a diet low in fat, and you're avoiding processed foods. But before you decide that a cave in the hills would make a lovely home for you and your family, let's move forward 30,000 years to the present.

The time we now live in is an era of information and technology. And in spite of some of the problems this technology has brought us, it has also provided us with some wonderful tools that our Cro-Magnon ancestors never had. Some of the most important of these advances have taken place in the field of medicine.

In this chapter, I'm going to tell you about the medical tools at your disposal that will aid you in staying healthy. Specifically, I'll talk about how early screening for cancer and heart disease can greatly improve your chances of surviving these illnesses.

Screening for Cancer and Heart Disease

One of the fundamental rules of medicine and good health is that early diagnosis of just about any illness is of great benefit to fighting the disease. This is especially true of cancer.

Remember that cancer doesn't take hold instantly. It passes through many phases, gradually accumulating more and more genetic damage to the cells until it finally takes over the body. So if cancer can be diagnosed early, most people have an excellent chance of surviving it.

Cancer of the cervix is probably the most striking example of how beneficial early diagnosis can be. Before the widespread use of the Pap smear, hundreds of thousands of women died of this cancer each year. Now that we know the importance of routine gynecological check-ups, that number is down to 4,500 each year. If *every* woman were to get routine Pap smears, the number of new cases would be close to zero.

In countries where screening is not accessible, most cancer victims don't see a doctor until the disease has reached an incurable stage. In India, for example, cervical cancer is the number-one cause of death among women.

Risk Assessment

We've developed a huge battery of devices, tests, and machines to help us diagnose cancer early. This is great news, but the truth is, it's a waste of time and money to screen every person for every conceivable type of disease. Screening should take place in a directed way—that is, those who are at risk should be tested. So if you don't smoke, it's usually not necessary to test you for lung cancer. Or if you're a woman in your 20s, you don't need regular mammograms (because breast cancer is extremely rare among young people).

So how do you determine what types of disease you are at risk for? A thorough explanation is beyond the scope of this book, but it is absolutely necessary for you to know your personal risk profile. Your physician should be able to provide you with this information based on your lifestyle, habits, family history, nutrition, prior medical history, and occupation. You may also find self-assessment risk evaluation tests in health and lifestyle magazines or in the form of computer software. Some health insurance companies also have risk assessment tools available.

Screening Techniques

Screening examinations specifically look for a disease in its earliest, and most curable, stage. Screening examinations come in all varieties, from the most simple (physical examination) to the most complex (polymerase chain reaction analysis of genes or gene products). Which screening techniques are suitable for you will depend on what cancers you are at risk for, how great your risk is, and the technology that is available.

Deciding which screening tests you may or may not need is best left to you and your doctor. But for your information, the following are several commonly available diagnostic techniques:

Physical examination: This is the simplest of all screening techniques and also the *least accurate*. Other than detecting cancers that can be easily felt or seen (such as breast or skin cancer), physical examination is a crude method of screening. Usually doctors couple this exam with other more advanced techniques.

Imaging studies: These x-ray and related procedures have come into widespread use in the past 20 years. We have made enormous advances in our ability to see inside the human body without cutting it open. Several commonly used imaging studies include:

- *Mammography*—Using this technique, breast cancers smaller than a grape seed can be regularly detected. Mammography has made a revolution in the early diagnosis of this disease.

- *CAT (Computer-Assisted Tomography) scans*—This technique has enabled doctors to look inside the human body with amazing clarity. The major disadvantage is that CAT scans expose the individual to radiation. (However, technological advances have significantly decreased x-ray doses, while faster computers have enhanced our ability to rapidly scan and quickly image any part of the body.)

❋ *MRI (Magnetic Resonance Imaging)*—This is a substantial leap beyond CAT scans because MRI uses no radiation. Instead, images are constructed by passing a strong magnetic field through the body and then "listening" to the "noise" created as molecules in cells change position in response to this field. A potential side effect: It has the ability to demagnetize your credit cards, so be sure to leave them at home!

❋ *Ultrasound*—In these examinations, high-frequency waves are passed through the body. The echo of the sound is detected, and a computer constructs a picture of the area. Ultrasound can be very helpful in differentiating between solid tumors and cysts (especially in breast examinations) and in imaging women's reproductive organs (the ovaries and the uterus).

❋ *Nuclear medicine scanning*—This technique uses trace (and essentially harmless) amounts of radioactive isotopes. It's especially helpful in detecting cancers in the thyroid, liver, and bones.

❋ *PET* (Positron Emission Tomography) scans—These are not commonly available and can only be obtained at specialized centers. However, this very useful technique is based on the way localized areas of the body metabolize sugar and other substances.

Cytology: This is the study of cells under the microscope. Looking at a Pap smear, pathologists and cytology technicians are able to differentiate between normal and cancerous cells. Keep in mind that the Pap smear is not just a test for cancer of the cervix. Any tissue specimen can be subjected to a Pap test. For instance, sputum cytology (a lung cancer test) and urine cytology (a test for bladder cancer) are also performed this way.

Biologic Markers: Many tumors make substances that leak into the bloodstream. Testing for the presence of these substances is a fairly accurate way of detecting certain types of cancer. For instance, finding increased levels of PSA (prostate-specific antigen) in the blood may indicate cancer of the prostate. CEA (carcinoembryonic antigen) is made by cancers of the intestines and some lung cancers. Other markers show up in cancers of the pancreas, ovaries, breast, lungs, intestines, and testicles.

Genetic markers: Scientists are now able to analyze DNA to assess a person's risk for a disease before it even occurs. These genetic tests have raised some ethical questions that are being wrestled with by professionals and advocacy groups. I take no sides here, but simply inform you that these tests exist. They are often performed to detect hereditary risk for breast cancer, cancer of the ovary, and cancer of the large intestine. A recent discovery is the breast cancer gene that puts women at high risk for breast AND ovarian cancer (see Table 11A below).

TABLE 11A

RISK OF CANCER OF THE BREAST AND OVARY
IN WOMEN WITH THE BREAST/OVARY CANCER GENE
(BRCA1)

Age	% Breast Cancer	% Ovarian Cancer	% Both
30	3	0	3
40	19	1	20
50	51	22	62
60	54	30	68
70	85	63	95

Adapted from: Easton DF, Ford BP, Bishop DT, and the Breast Cancer Linkage Consortium; Am. J. Hum. Genet. 56:265, 1995.

Screening for Specific Cancers

Once your doctor has determined your personal risk profile, he or she will probably recommend that you be screened for one or more specific cancers. Types of cancers that can be screened for include:

Breast cancer: *(Risk factors: diet [high fat], family history, early menarche, late menopause, first full-term pregnancy after age 33)* There is no question that mammograms performed on a routine basis for women over 50 are highly effective in diagnosing and curing these lesions. But a controversy exists as to whether women under 50 should undergo these screenings. Personally, I encourage them. Researchers and public policy makers have to weigh the risks against the global costs of these techniques. Currently, the American Cancer Society recommends that women receive mammograms every other year between the ages of 40 to 50 and every year beginning after age 50. Women who are at particularly high risk because of family history are encouraged to have yearly screenings beginning earlier.

The simplest, most cost-effective, and easiest screening test for breast cancer is breast self-examination. This test is free, can be accomplished at home, and can be done frequently (at least once a month). Statistically 80 to 90 percent of all palpable breast lumps are found by patients on their own. Mammography is best suited to detect breast cancers that are too small to be felt.

To graphically see the relationship between breast cancer and fat intake, I have included Table 11B, which looks at fat intake internationally.

Table 11B

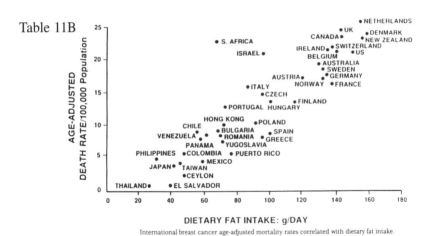

International breast cancer age-adjusted mortality rates correlated with dietary fat intake.

Cervical cancer: (*Risk factors: having multiple sex partners, infection with papilloma virus*) In general, women are advised to get Pap smears every year. However, yearly screenings may be too frequent for many women. Many medical professionals recommend that if a woman in her early 20s has three normal Pap smears (each taken a year apart), screening frequency can be reduced to every two or three years. I urge you to talk with your doctor about this.

Cancer of the uterus: *(Risk factors: diet [high-fat], obesity, diabetes).* This cancer is screened for during pelvic examinations and Pap smears. Once again, I recommend that women have these exams yearly or as otherwise advised by their gynecologist.

Cancer of the ovary: *(Risk factors: diet [high-fat], never having been pregnant, family history)* Screening for ovarian cancer is still in its infancy. Ultrasound, a physical exam, and a blood test can be used, but the sensitivity and specificity are low. It is generally not necessary for women at normal risk to undergo these screenings.

Colon cancer: *(Risk factors: diet high in red meat, family history, presence of polyps in the colon. Protective factors: daily dose of aspirin, high-fiber diet, green leafy vegetables)* Cancer of the large intestine is fairly common. The good news is that it can be detected in several different ways while it is still in a curable stage. The simplest screening technique is testing stools for blood. This test is so fast and easy to do that every adult over the age of 35 should have this screening performed on a yearly basis.

However, colon cancer in a very early stage may not have grown large enough to bleed, so doctors must look directly at the inside of the large intestine. This is accomplished using either a sigmoidoscope or a colonoscope. This test used to be accomplished using rigid tubes, but as a result of recent scientific advances, these tubes are now bendable fiber optic scopes. The procedure is slightly uncomfortable but not painful.

Both scopes are similar in function; however, a sigmoidoscope can see only the lower part of the large intestine, while a colonoscope can view the entire colon. For this reason, I feel that use of a colonoscope is more effective. Why take a chance of missing a cancer because the scope can't reach it?

For those of us at normal risk, either a colonoscopy or sigmoidoscopy should be performed every few years beginning at age 50.

Cancer of the testicles: *(Risk factor: undescended testicle at birth)* This cancer is rare but can be easily diagnosed by the patient. The cancer tends to occur in the teens and twenties. Young men at risk are advised to do testicular self-examinations. (Ask your doctor for more information.)

Skin cancer: *(Risk factors: heavy sun exposure, history of blistering* *sunburn, fair skin, blond hair)* There are no technologically advanced screening tests for this cancer other than routine skin examinations. At-risk individuals should perform self-exams and have examinations performed by their doctors.

Lung cancer: (*Risk factors: smoking, smoking, and smoking! Other factors include chronic lung disease, diet, and some occupations. Protective factors: never smoking, eating foods containing vitamin A)* Screening for lung cancer is a controversial area. There is evidence that blanket screening of a population is neither biologically sound nor cost-effective. However, smokers over 55 who have symptoms of chronic lung disease (cough, phlegm production, emphysema) may undergo a chest x-ray combined with a Pap smear of lung secretions. More sensitive screening tests will be available soon.

Cancer of the prostate: (*Risk factors: diet [high fat], being African-American, having multiple sex partners. This cancer also may be correlated with infection by the papilloma virus.)* The prostate is the organ in males that adds a liquid medium in which sperm are mixed. The prostate is attached to the bottom of the bladder in front of the rectum about three to four inches from the anus. The prostate can be felt during a rectal examination. This test, coupled with the PSA blood test, are important for individuals over age 45, who should have these tests performed every year.

Cancer of the bladder: (*Risk factors: Smoking is the greatest risk factor. Other factors include diet and certain occupations.)* Simple tests such as urine analysis (looking for blood) and a Pap smear of urine specimen cells are good screenings for the early detection of bladder cancer. Other methods will soon be available. If you are at risk, your doctor will advise you how often these tests should be performed.

Early Diagnosis (Screening) and Heart Disease

There is a commonly held belief that heart disease is a "kinder and gentler" ailment than cancer. This is simply not true. Those who have been diagnosed with heart disease have about the same chance of surviving as those who have contracted cancer. However, much like cancer, early detection of heart problems will lead to improved end results. Screening for *any killer disease makes a big difference*, and heart disease is no exception.

The silver standard for screening is the treadmill stress test. During the test, a person's cardiogram is recorded while he or she walks at a rapid pace on the treadmill. If there is a significant problem with blood supply to the heart muscle, it is readily detected. This test can be combined with nuclear medicine and ultrasound techniques to further refine interpretation of the results.

This test is recommended for all at-risk individuals beginning by age 40.

A Final Word of Caution

Screening for heart disease and cancer can prolong your life and keep you healthy. However, please remember that no screening test is 100 percent foolproof. All screening tests have occasional false-negative and false-positive results. For this reason, screening tests should probably not be undertaken unless risk factors are present. I urge you to discuss this issue with your health-care provider.

❊ ❊ ❊ ❊ ❊ ❊

Chapter Twelve

The Evolutionary Diet — Your Chance to Live a Long and Healthy Life

Most of us cringe at the mere mention of the word *diet*. It conjures up images of dreary meals—small, dreary meals. Personally, I picture a large plate with a small carrot in the middle, decorated with a sprig of parsley.

The *Oxford American Dictionary's* second definition of the word *diet* is "a severe restriction." However, the first definition is not nearly as unpleasant: "The sort of foods eaten by a person or community." And that is how I like to refer to the word *diet* in this book. The Evolutionary Diet is about cooking and eating the sort of foods that are good for us genetically—foods eaten by a community that is in sync with its environment.

The Plan: Putting It All Together

Now that you have a relatively solid understanding of the principles of Evolutionary eating, let me give you some tips on putting the diet into practice in your everyday life.

#1: Don't Count Calories

The reality is, counting calories is not the best way to lose weight. Monitoring the calories for every bite of food you put into your mouth is time-consuming and often more trouble than it's worth. So why did I include a table of calories for weight maintenance and list calorie amounts for each recipe? Because being *aware* of calories (especially fat calories) is very important. And you can easily educate yourself by spending a few weeks looking at labels and caloric values of recipes. After a very short while, you will comfortably recognize the foods that are high in calories and especially high in saturated fats. Most of them are obvious. We all know a piece of chocolate cake a la mode is one of those things to avoid, as is a hamburger and fries.

#2: Get 25 Percent or Less of Your Calories from Fat

Cutting your fat intake to a moderate 25 percent is not that difficult to achieve. Once again, if you educate yourself by reading labels in the super-market, you will quickly get a sense of how to eat a low-fat diet.

#3: Eat More Unsaturated Than Saturated Fat

Always eat more unsaturated fat than saturated fat. Remember, satu-rated fat is the kind that hardens at room temperature. This includes butter, lard, cheese, and most animal fat. Unsaturated fat is found in vegetable oils (such as olive, peanut, and canola). Even though it's considered "the good fat," unsaturated fat should still be consumed in small quantities. (Remember, you're trying to keep your total fat intake at around 25 percent of calories.)

#4: Get 25 Percent of Your Calories from Protein

Getting 25 percent of your calories from protein is much higher than recommended by several "high-carbohydrate diet gurus." But recent stud-ies show that despite the growing health awareness in the United States, we are still getting fatter. In fact, about a third of our population is obese. High-carbohydrate diets are partly to blame. They don't work because our 30,000-year-old genes need more protein.

Good sources of protein are wild game, fish, shellfish, and skinless poultry. Also don't forget nuts and legumes (beans are about 30 percent protein).

#5: Get 50 Percent of Your Calories from Carbohydrates

This is easy. Fruits, vegetables, grains, and legumes are all very high in carbohydrates. Have an extra vegetable for dinner. Your fat calories will be lower, and you won't be hungry.

#6: Eat Only Nonfat Dairy Products

Once you're weaned as an infant, you don't need any more dairy. You do need vitamin D and calcium, but you can get these nutrients from other foods. If you don't want to forsake dairy completely, you can consume nonfat dairy products. Remember, though, that *low*-fat is really a misnomer. Most low-fat dairy foods are actually high in fat. So stick to nonfat for good health.

#7: Don't Worry About Cholesterol

You can eat as much cholesterol-rich food as you want and still have a healthy heart—as long as your diet is low in saturated fat. So go ahead and enjoy high-cholesterol lobster, crab, shrimp, scallops, clams, and mussels; just don't dip them, bread them, or fry them in butter.

#8: Eat Lots of Fiber

Fiber plays several important roles in keeping us healthy. It reduces the risk for heart disease and several types of cancer. It also adds bulk to the diet without adding any calories. Make fruits, vegetables, and grains a regular part of your diet—your body will tell you when you're eating enough.

#9: Eat Very Little Salt

Start reducing the quantity of salt in your diet by not salting your food when you sit down to a meal. Some restaurants don't even have salt shakers on the tables! When cooking, remember that salt should only be added to bring out the natural flavors of the food, not to mask them. You can use other spices and condiments in place of salt and still get the same enjoyment out of your meal.

#10: Take a Baby Aspirin Every Day (with Your Doctor's Permission)

This simple addition to your daily routine can reduce your risk of heart disease and colon cancer significantly.

#11: Get Appropriate Health Screenings

Eating correctly is the first way to avoid cancer and heart disease. The second step is learning what diseases you are at risk for and catching any abnormalities early. Cancers that are cured are those that are caught in the earliest stages; similarly, early diagnosis of coronary heart disease significantly decreases your chance of premature death. Once again, a healthy diet should be followed no matter what your other risk factors may be.

#12: Exercise Often

Even if your time is limited, you can still reap the benefits of exercise. Walking every day (say, before or after dinner) will keep you healthier than running a marathon every month.

#13: Affirm to Yourself Every Day That You Deserve to Be Healthy and Live a Long Life

Setting a goal of good health is the first step to achieving it. Tell yourself on a daily basis that you deserve a healthy, attractive body, and you'll find it easier to begin Evolutionary eating.

#14: Feed Your Children a Hunter-Gatherer Diet

After you've put the principles of the Evolutionary Diet to work in your own life, share your new, healthful habits with your children. By eating responsibly (low-fat, not no-fat) while you're pregnant (and breast-feeding), and by feeding your children responsibly after they're weaned, you're providing them with a jump start to a long life free of cancer and heart disease.

#15: Occasionally Break the Rules

If you watch your fat intake carefully, you can splurge occasionally and have something very high in fat. However, as you begin eating the Evolutionary Diet, I think you'll find that your cravings for foods high in saturated fat will diminish, and that over time, a steak will taste so heavy and rich, you won't want to eat very much of it.

Summary: The 15 Guidelines to a Long and Healthy Life

Once you begin the Evolutionary Diet, you'll find that it is, in fact, very easy to follow. Stick to the 15 guidelines of the plan, and you will lose weight, look and feel better, and live longer.

1. DON'T COUNT CALORIES.
2. GET 25 PERCENT OR LESS OF YOUR CALORIES FROM FAT.
3. EAT MORE UNSATURATED FAT THAN SATURATED.
4. GET 25 PERCENT OF YOUR CALORIES FROM PROTEIN.
5. GET 50 PERCENT OF YOUR CALORIES FROM CARBOHYDRATES.
6. EAT ONLY NONFAT DAIRY FOODS.
7. DON'T WORRY ABOUT CHOLESTEROL.
8. EAT LOTS OF FIBER.
9. EAT VERY LITTLE SALT.
10. TAKE A BABY ASPIRIN EVERY DAY.
11. GET APPROPRIATE HEALTH SCREENINGS.
12. EXERCISE OFTEN.
13. AFFIRM TO YOURSELF EVERY DAY THAT YOU DESERVE TO BE HEALTHY AND LIVE A LONG LIFE.
14. FEED YOUR CHILDREN A HUNTER-GATHERER DIET.
15. OCCASIONALLY BREAK THE RULES.

Now, we recommend that you read these guidelines again, write them down or copy this page from the book, and carry them with you until they become part of your *personal evolution.*

❊ ❊ ❊ ❊ ❊ ❊

PART II
Eating for Health and Enjoyment

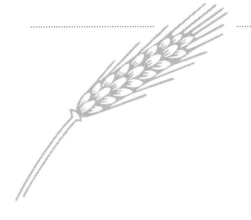

Chapter Thirteen

The Joys of Food

(I have asked Kathye to share in the writing of this chapter, so if you notice one of us referring to the other, it's because there are two voices at work here.)

Food and Love *(According to Ron)*

"Do you love me?" I asked, as the pasta overcooked. "Yes, I will love you forever," Kathye replied. And that is, sort of, kind of, how Kathye and I met and fell in love. She had been chef-owner of a successful catering firm, host of a radio cooking show, and a popular cooking teacher. I had worked in professional kitchens and had spent much of my free time sampling new recipes. Food was the first topic we had in common.

Today, Kathye and I celebrate our lives together and our love for one another partially through the preparation and enjoyment of food. We are two peas in a pod. She is my Parvati and I am her Shiva (Hindu gods who were such great partners that they became one). That is, the composite of us both is more than the sum of our parts when it comes to many things, cooking being one of them.

For us, food is much more than something that sustains our health; food is a way of celebrating life. Many of my good memories of childhood are centered around food. I can still smell the turkey roasting in my mother's kitchen on Thanksgiving Day and the smell of the hamburgers and hot dogs grilling on the barbeque on the 4th of July.

Food has played a large role in my adult life as well. At birthdays and births, reunions and unions, welcomes and farewells, my loved ones and I have come together, shared in each other's company, and raised our forks and glasses to one another.

For Kathye and me, joy and happiness are integral parts of cooking and cuisine. We hope to share this pleasure with you by introducing you to some new ways of preparing food that will bring you both culinary pleasure and good health.

The First Dinner (According to Kathye)

The first time Ron invited me to dinner, he asked me if there were any foods I didn't like or didn't eat. Considering myself very sophisticated in the area of cuisine, I said out loud that I wasn't crazy about jellyfish and added silently to myself, "Or sea urchin." Of course, one of the courses he served would have to include a sea urchin sauce. (See recipe for Shiitake Open-Faced Sandwiches on page 177.) But the real surprise for me was that the sauce was delicious!

Since then, Ron has changed the whole way I look at food. In this section of the book, we hope you'll learn to broaden your culinary interests. And by learning a few cooking tricks, you won't even notice that you've reduced the fat in your diet. But you *will* notice that you're getting healthier, thinner, and having more fun.

The Noble Carrot

Part of the reason why Kathye and I love to cook and eat is diversity. We live in a city (Los Angeles) where 103 languages are spoken, and the variety of foods is endless. This means that we can eat healthily while still enjoying foods rich in flavor. Let me give you an example of how we do so.

Start with a food that's very good for you, such as a carrot. A raw carrot doesn't sound very exciting, but now begin to think of this carrot dressed, not naked. That same carrot as part of a gazpacho, or caramelized to accompany roast chicken, starts to look very different. If you cook a carrot with some rosemary and oregano in a little bit of olive oil, it takes on an Italian flavor. With dates and raisins, a carrot turns into a side dish at a Moroccan meal. Cooked in coriander, cumin, and turmeric, the carrot ends up being an Indian-style dish. With a little bacon (just enough for the smoky taste), onions, and apples, carrots turn German. Carrots with garlic, soy sauce, sesame oil, rice wine vinegar, and Szechwan peppercorns taste Chinese. Take the same lowly carrot and cook it with some ginger and non-fat sour cream, and its Russian flavor will come out. Try stir-frying carrots with shallots, turmeric, peanut butter, sugar, and vinegar to make carrots with an Indonesian touch. An ancient Roman way of cooking carrots is adding wine, vegetable stock, olive oil, and ground pepper. Turkish carrots? Sure! Add olive oil, caraway seeds, and nonfat yogurt. And finally, a perfect Pakistani dessert: a carrot pudding with nonfat milk, saffron, ground almonds, sugar, and cardamon. And this is just using a carrot as an example. Think of what you can do with fish or fowl!

The recipes in the cookbook section draw on the Noble Carrot principle to make cooking and eating more fun. Once you start experimenting with some different (sometimes exotic) ingredients, you'll marvel at the wide variety of delicious foods you are able to prepare. And you won't even notice that you're eating less fat. (We have included a list of mail-order resources for foreign ingredients in case you can't get them locally.)

What Country Would You Like to Eat in Tonight?

To illustrate the way we think about food, listed below is a week's worth of menus from around the world, all healthy and delicious and full of flavor. (At this point, just read them over to get a feel for the types of foods the Evolutionary Diet consists of. You'll find some of the recipes following this chapter.) These menus show how it's possible to cook in any style by starting with a main ingredient and then changing either the cooking method or the spices (the Noble Carrot principle). If there are ingredients you simply don't like, leave them out. But we encourage you to try everything. You might even find, as Kathye did, that sea urchin is great!

The Italian Evolutionary Diet

Lunch

PASTA SALAD
Served warm or cold with tomato and lots of fresh herbs
such as tarragon, basil, and thyme.

Dinner

MEDITERRANEAN CHICKEN
With grilled bell peppers, onions, garlic, tomatoes, and
olives and simmered slowly like a stew.

VEGETABLE RISOTTO
ORANGE AND MINT SALAD

The Chinese Evolutionary Diet

Lunch

STEAMED FISH
With ginger, garlic, soy sauce, and parsley.

STEAMED RICE AND DAIKON RADISH SALAD

Dinner

STIR-FRIED CHICKEN
With cilantro

GREEN SALAD WITH SWEET AND SOUR DRESSING

The Indian Evolutionary Diet

Lunch

SPICY CHICKEN SOUP
Made with potatoes and aromatic Eastern spices
such as cumin and coriander

RAITA
A salad with yogurt, cucumber, and red onion

Dinner

TOMATO AND ONION SALAD
With ginger tamarind dressing

CURRIED FISH
RICE WITH CARDAMON
BANANAS WITH HONEY AND YOGURT

The French Evolutionary Diet

Lunch

WARM DUCK BREAST SALAD
On a bed of lettuce with grilled morel mushrooms and green beans

Dinner

ROASTED VENISON
Marinated and grilled, served with chestnuts and baked apple

CELERY ROOT AND POTATO PUREE
FIGS MARINATED IN COGNAC

The Thai Evolutionary Diet

Lunch

LARB
Stir-fried chicken with fish sauce, chilies, lemon grass,
onion, and spices. Served on romaine leaves.

RAW VEGGIES (even carrots)

Dinner
SPICY MUSSELS
Cooked with ginger, chili, and garlic

THAI SHRIMP AND RICE NOODLE SALAD
With Napa cabbage and lime juice

The Vegetarian Evolutionary Diet

Lunch

THREE SALADS
Beets and cucumber with balsamic vinegar
Jicama with chives
Raisins, carrots, walnuts, and yogurt

Dinner

GRILLED PORTOBELLO MUSHROOMS
PASTA SALAD WITH EGGPLANT
DATE AND APPLE MOUSSE

The American Evolutionary Diet

Lunch

POACHED SQUID WITH BLACK BEANS
WATERCRESS, FENNEL, AND ENDIVE SALAD

Dinner

GRILLED SALMON
With tomatillo salsa

OKRA IN LOUISIANA SPICES
GRAPE SHERBET

A Few Words about Breakfast

For decades, we have eaten a morning repast that is unique to the United States. It's a big breakfast of bacon, eggs, fried potatoes, pancakes, and so on—in other words, one filled with saturated fat. The rationale has been that a hearty breakfast will give us the energy to get up and go. But the reverse may well be true: starting the day with a diet high in protein and low in fat may be the healthiest thing we can do.

In many countries, breakfast is a variation on the other meals of the day. The Japanese eat a healthy morning meal consisting of fish, rice, and vegetables. This breakfast is very high in protein, low in fat, and tastes remarkably good. It's energy-rich and low in fat and sugar. However, eating rice and fish may not be practical for you. If that's the case, try modifying your typical breakfast: Substitute nonfat milk for regular milk, cereal for eggs, and fruit in place of potatoes (although the potatoes are fine if they're made without fat).

A bran muffin may be tasty and filling, but beware of its contents and avoid those made with saturated fats. The same is true of cereal; read the labels carefully and avoid those containing sugar.

Before You Turn on the Stove...

A few tips before you start washing, chopping, and tossing food on the fire:

- ※ **Buy a variety of cookbooks.** Cookbooks are wonderful teachers and great resources. By looking through a variety of different recipes, you will begin to get a feel for the wide range of ways to cook a carrot or an onion or a fish or a bird or whatever. This is when the "Where Do I Want to Eat Tonight?" principle comes in.

- ※ **Keep the basic ingredients on hand.** By "basic ingredients," we don't mean the things you buy every day such as fresh chicken or fish; we mean the ingredients that are necessary to help you cook internationally. We have included an "International Basic Shopping List" for you later on in this chapter. Keep these items on hand, and then when you decide to have carrots or chicken, a world of possibilities awaits you. Remember, if you can't get some of the foreign foods locally, there is a mail-order resource list in the back of the book.

※ **Have the right tools available.** We have included a short list of tools that are valuable for healthy cooking at the end of this chapter, as well as some specialty items that come in handy when making more exotic recipes.

※ **To help keep your meals low in fat:**

1. Use nonstick pans for cooking—a good-quality pan makes a BIG difference.
2. When sauteing, spray first with PAM (Brand name) or any vegetable spray.
3. To scrupulously avoid extra fat, saute by adding vegetable juice (for example, tomato juice) and no oil. When the liquid has absorbed, cook until the ingredients have browned.
4. ALWAYS trim your meat of all the fat that you can see.

THE BASICS

Stock Can Make a Meal

In our opinion, there is nothing that makes more of a difference in the outcome of a main dish or sauce than the stock (broth) that is used, and we think that the top chefs all over the world would agree. Chicken, meat, and vegetable stocks are easy to make, but time-consuming to prepare. Fish stock is easy and takes very little time.

If you have a freezer, you can make a big, wonderful pot of stock and freeze it in small containers to use over many months. If it's impractical for you to make your own stock, buy nonfat, low-sodium chicken or vegetable broth at your local market. (The words *stock* and *broth* can be used interchangeably.)

The Basics

BASIC FISH STOCK

Prep Time: 15 minutes
Cook Time: 30 minutes

1 Tbsp. vegetable oil
2 lbs. fish bones including fish heads
   (except salmon), washed and chopped
1 large onion, chopped fine
4 stalks celery, chopped fine
1 leek, white part only, chopped fine
1 bay leaf
1 bunch (or less) parsley, chopped fine
$1/2$ cup white wine (optional)
water
$1/4$ tsp. salt
6 peppercorns

    In a stockpot, heat the oil over medium-high heat until quite hot. Add onions, celery, leeks, the bay leaf, parsley, and fish bones. Saute, stirring frequently, until the onions become translucent—about 5 minutes. Turn off the heat and allow to sit for 5 minutes.

    Add the wine, salt, pepper, and enough water to cover: about 8 cups. Bring to a boil uncovered, and skim any foam off the surface as the mixture begins to boil. Reduce heat and continue cooking for 20 to 30 minutes. Skim the surface occasionally, when foam or scum rises to the top. Remove from the heat and strain. When cool, the stock can be refrigerated for several days or frozen for later use.

Makes about 6–8 cups

Shortcut: A simple shellfish stock can be made by boiling the shells of any shellfish with a sliced onion in water for as little as 10 minutes. The results are much better than just using water. You can also substitute a small bottle of clam juice, a cup of dry vermouth, and a cup of water.

The Basics

BASIC VEGETABLE STOCK

Easy

Prep Time: 15 minutes
Cook Time: 1 hour, 20 minutes

      2 onions, thinly chopped
      2 cloves garlic, crushed
      1 leek, white part only, cleaned and chopped
      2 carrots, chopped
      1–2 potatoes, thinly sliced
      2 stalks celery, sliced
      6 sprigs parsley, coarsely chopped
      6 sprigs thyme
      3 oregano sprigs
      3 marjoram sprigs
      2 bay leaves
      1 tsp. salt
      1-2 black peppercorns
      9–10 cups cold water

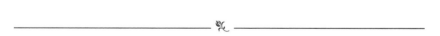

In a large stockpot, heat water. Add the onion, leek, garlic, and salt. Stir for 2 minutes, then cover, and cook on medium heat for 15 minutes. Add all the other ingredients. Bring to a boil, reduce heat, and simmer (uncovered) for 60 minutes, skimming the surface frequently. Strain, pressing the vegetables to get as much liquid from them as possible. Discard the veggies. Freeze in pint-size containers for later use.

Makes 7–8 cups

The Basics

BASIC CHICKEN STOCK

Easy

Prep Time: 30 minutes
Cook Time: 2–10 hours

2 quarts (about 4 lbs.) of chicken pieces with bones
(chicken backs are great for this, although we usually
use a whole chicken as well).
1 Tbsp. oil
2 stalks celery, chopped
2 carrots, chopped
2 onions, chopped
1 Tbsp. fresh thyme, chopped
1 Tbsp. fresh oregano, chopped
2 cloves garlic, chopped
$1/2$ red chili, chopped (optional)
1 bay leaf
8 parsley stems
14–16 cups water

Chop the chicken, bones, and skin into 2"– 4" pieces (with a meat cleaver, if you have one). Brown in oil, stirring occasionally. Although the browning is not a required step, the result is a much richer, browner stock, and we think well worth the extra time. (If you're using your stock for making something light in color, such as potato leek soup, then skip the browning step.)

When the chicken is browned, add onion, celery, carrot, garlic, chili, thyme, and oregano. Cook on medium heat, stirring occasionally, until the vegetables color—about 5–10 minutes. Cover with water, and bring to a simmer. As the mixture simmers, gray scum, foam, and fat will rise to the surface. Skim it off occasionally until it ceases to rise. Cover the stockpot loosely, and allow to simmer for at least 2 hours, adding additional water if the liquid cooks down below the level of the other ingredients. For a really intense flavor, continue simmering, skimming, and adding water all day. Strain through a sieve into a bowl, and remove any remaining fat with a separator (degreaser). Allow to cool uncovered. Taste. If flavorful, refrigerate or freeze. If not, boil off some of the liquid to concentrate the stock.

Makes about 8 cups

Beans, Beans, the Wonderful Food

Beans and lentils are among the world's oldest foods and are full of protein. Most dried beans on the market need only one hour of soaking time, and if you have a pressure cooker, you can cook your beans or lentils in very little time.

One cup of dried beans produces 3 cups of cooked beans and serves 4–6. Canned beans of any type may be substituted for dried beans, but should be rinsed well before using.

BASIC RECIPE FOR ALL DRIED BEANS

Easy

Prep Time: 15 minutes
Cook Time: 1 to 2 hours, or 20 minutes if using a pressure cooker.

Two cups dried beans, rinsed and picked over to remove any small rocks or debris, then presoaked by boiling for 2 minutes in 6 or more cups of water, covered, removed from the heat and allowed to sit for one hour.

1 onion, chopped	1 carrot, chopped
1–2 cloves garlic, chopped	2 cloves
2" of ham hock or other salt	parsley
pork (optional)	6–8 cups water

Rinse the beans after soaking and add to a large saucepan with all the other ingredients. Simmer, partially covered, for 1–2 hours until tender. Remove any fat that rises to the top from the ham hock. Allow the beans to cool in their cooking liquid, then cover and refrigerate. Can be made two days ahead.

To cook in a pressure cooker, follow the pressure cooker instructions. We use 15 lbs. pressure for 3 minutes, and then let the pressure go down for at least 10–15 minutes before uncovering.

Makes 6 cups beans

Herbs and Spices

If you can get them or grow them, fresh herbs really are delicious. They will lose some of their flavor if cooked for a long period of time. So, always add a few extra pinches as you serve the dish. Dried herbs are more intense than fresh ones. If you're using dried herbs in a recipe calling for fresh herbs, use about half as much. The bottom line is to trust your taste buds. If there is not enough flavor of an herb you like, add more. If you're concerned that the recipe calls for too much, add half the amount, taste after the dish has cooked for a while, then add more to your taste.

Frying spices in a skillet for 15 seconds to a minute will release their aroma and flavor. Grinding your own spices (in a little grinder like a coffee mill) will give you a fresher, more aromatic spice.

A Word about "Heat"

If variety is the spice of life, chilies will add spice to your preparations in almost infinite variety, too. You will notice that in some of the recipes we have added the ingredient "heat" without further comment. The reason for this is that you may have some particular preference or aversion to some or all of the "hot" ingredients. For instance, there are individuals who do not add anything made from peppers to their food. These people can add heat in other forms such as ground black peppercorns.

Remember, you are not adding just heat, but flavor as well. The taste of a Szechwan peppercorn, white peppercorn, black peppercorn, or pink peppercorn is quite different. Similarly, the chilies come in great variety from sweet and mild to fiery hot. But they too have a flavor separate from the heat. We suggest that you experiment with many of them. Personally we use mostly black and white pepper, habanero, serrano, chipotle, jalapeno, and pascilla chilies. The other heats, such as Szechwan and pink peppercorns, are used in exotic preparations, and we have not included recipes with these ingredients.

How to Keep a Larder Without Lard

If you keep nonperishable ingredients on hand, using the Evolutionary Diet recipes will be easy. However, check your pantry to be sure the items are low in fat. Discard **ALL** your butter and dairy products (except those that are nonfat), as well as any canned goods (such as broth) that are high in fat. Next, go to the market (when you're not hungry) and shop for nonfat nonperishables.

A Larder of All the Basics for the Evolutionary Recipes

Don't forget, what is unavailable locally can be ordered from one of the sources in the Glossary. The Glossary also includes a description of unusual and foreign ingredients.

<u>Beans, Rice, and Grains</u>

black beans, dried or canned	basmati rice
great northern beans, dried or canned	bulgur wheat
fava beans, dried or canned	couscous
garbanzo beans, canned	lentils
brown rice	pearl barley
arborio rice	pearl pasta (Israeli couscous)
corn meal	quinoa

<u>Dried Herbs and Spices Probably Available at Your Local Market</u>

basil	bay leaves	cardamom	caraway seeds
cayenne pepper	celery seed	chervil	chili powder
chives	cilantro	cinnamon	cloves
coriander seed	cumin	cumin (ground)	curry powder
dill	fennel	ginger powder	five spice
mint	garlic powder	allspice	powder (Chinese)

More Dried Herbs and Spices

mustard seed	dry mustard	nutmeg	onion
oregano	paprika	parsley	black pepper
rosemary	poultry seasoning	saffron	sesame seeds
salt (Kosher)	dried shallots	tarragon	thyme
turmeric	vanilla		

Oils and Vinegars

apple cider	balsamic vinegar	red wine vinegar
rice wine vinegar	raspberry vinegar	white wine vinegar
chili oil	olive oil	peanut oil
sesame oil	truffle oil	walnut oil
mustard oil	vegetable oil	canola oil

Dried or Canned Chilies and Mushrooms
(may not be available at your market)

Anaheim or New Mexico chilies	chipotle chilies (canned)
habanera chili	jalapeno chilies (canned)
red chilies (in spice section)	pascilla chilies
morel mushrooms (dried)	shiitake mushrooms (Japanese)

Sugars and Liquors

sugar	Kahlua	mirin (also called
brown sugar	Pernod	aji-mirin, sweet
molasses	maple syrup	cooking rice
honey	cognac or brandy	wine of Japan)
bourbon	sake (Japanese)	

Sauces and Condiments

capers	catsup	chili sauce
horseradish	mushroom soy sauce (Chinese)	pickle relish
soy sauce	Tabasco	Dijon mustard
Worcestershire sauce	lime juice	lemon juice
clam juice		

Canned, Boxed, and Frozen Basics

nonfat low-sodium chicken broth	nonfat vegetable broth
evaporated skim milk	black olives
sundried tomato paste	tomato paste
water chestnuts, canned	pumpkin
frozen corn	frozen peas
frozen blueberries	raisins
dried fruits	dark chocolate
canned lychee nuts (Chinese)	smoked ham hock
canned grape leaves (Middle Eastern)	

Asian Specialty Items
(may not be available at your market)

bean sauce	fermented black beans	bonito
fish sauce	galanga	lemon grass
oyster sauce	Hoisin sauce	miso
rice noodles	rice sticks	shrimp paste
wasabi	dried shiitake mushrooms	yamagobo
mushroom soy	dried seaweed	star anise

Indian Specialty Items
(may not be available at your market)

asafetida	kabob spice paste	tikka paste
tamarind	fenugreek	

Middle Eastern
(may not be available at your market)

harissa   grape leaves

A Few Tools to Make Your Life As a Chef Easier

These are a few things you may not already have in your kitchen that make a difference in healthy cooking:

- Blender or food processor
- Small grinder for spices and coffee
- Two nonstick skillets, one small and one large (we have found that investing in good-quality nonstick pans is well worth the expense. They don't scratch easily, are heavy enough to cook evenly, and really don't stick.)
- Wok—great for quick cooking with very little oil and can double as a smoker
- Separator (or degreaser)—so you can easily get rid of any extra fat
- A Sharp Knife

On to the Recipes

On the following pages, you will find about 150 recipes. They are divided into categories such as "QUICK and EASY" (for those of you who don't have the interest or time for extensive cooking), "ADVENTUR-OUS," and others. All are compatible with your genes as well as your taste buds. We hope you enjoy them, along with your new, healthy life.

❈ ❈ ❈ ❈ ❈ ❈

Chapter Fourteen

The Recipes

The recipes are divided into:

❋ **QUICK AND EASY**
These are recipes that can be easily substituted for fast foods.

❋ **EASY**
These are recipes that are not complicated but take a little longer to prepare than those that are QUICK AND EASY.

❋ **QUICK AND ADVENTUROUS**
These recipes have a short preparation time but may have foreign or unusual ingredients. A description of each of these ingredients can be found in the Glossary. For those of you who can't find these ingredients in your local markets or specialty stores, we have also included a list of specialty stores and mail-order sources to assist you.

❋ **ADVENTUROUS**
These recipes are for those of you who really like cooking and are willing and/or able to spend a little extra time to create a memorable meal.

CHEFS' NOTE

The calories per serving listed with each recipe are approximate and meant to act as a guide for you. They were computed using the combination of a computer program and data from nutritional labels. In a few cases of foreign or exotic ingredients (for example, sea urchin ["uni"]), we have estimated caloric value from our knowledge of the food. Although we believe these caloric values to be accurate, we cannot accept responsibility for errors in the computer program or inaccurate data received from food producers or sellers.

All of our recipes are low in saturated fat.

(see recipe on page 172)

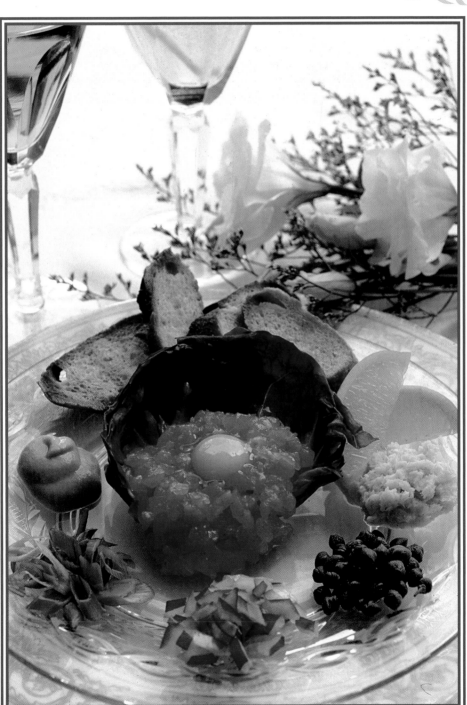

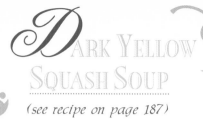

Dark Yellow Squash Soup

(see recipe on page 187)

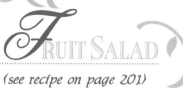

Fruit Salad

(see recipe on page 201)

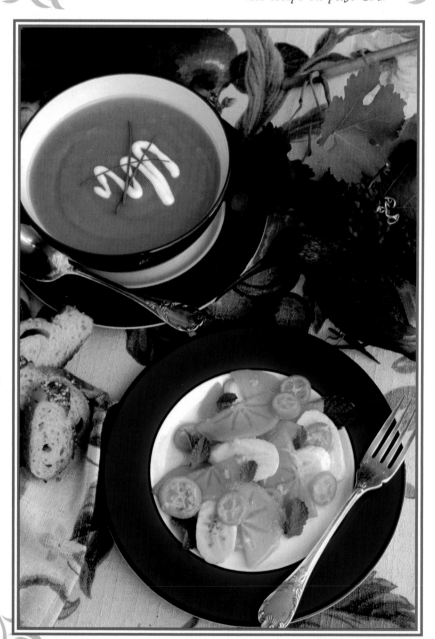

Setting courtesy of Crate and Barrel

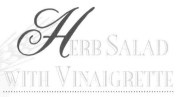

WILD MUSHROOM SANDWICH ON CARAWAY POLENTA TOAST

(see recipe on page 226)

HERB SALAD WITH VINAIGRETTE

(use your favorite vinaigrette)

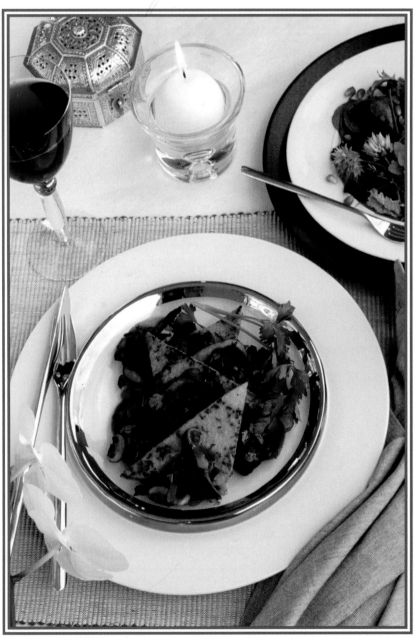

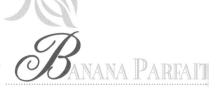
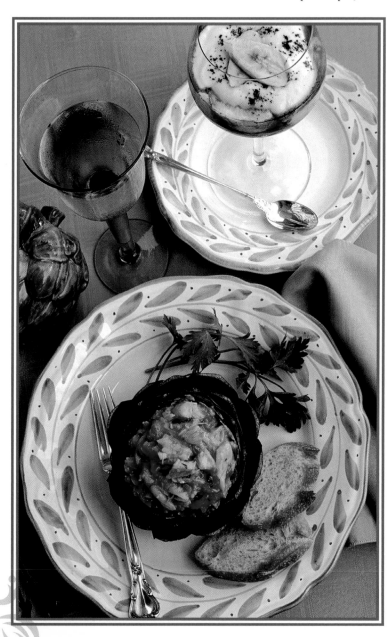

"TWO CUP" MUSHROOM BARLEY SOUP

(see recipe on page 186)

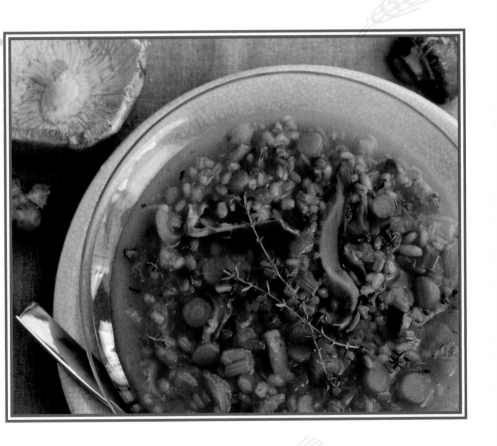

Roasted Turkey Sandwich with BBQ Sauce and Creamy Slaw

(see recipes on pages 272, 315, 200)

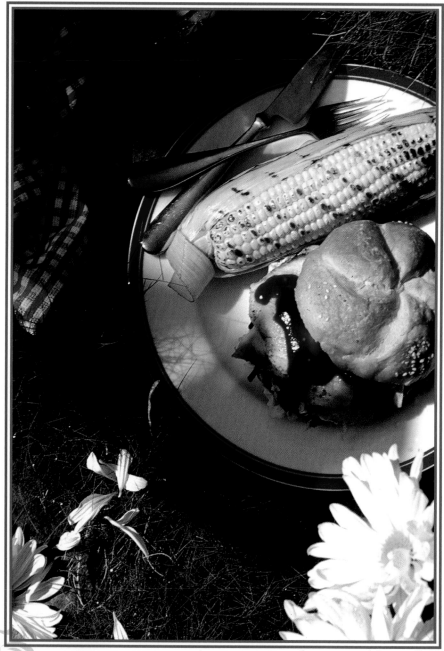

Setting courtesy of Crate and Barrel

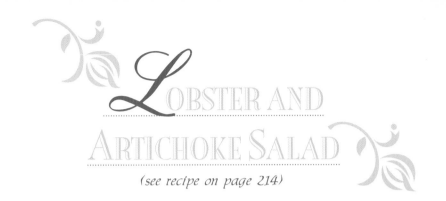

LOBSTER AND ARTICHOKE SALAD

(see recipe on page 214)

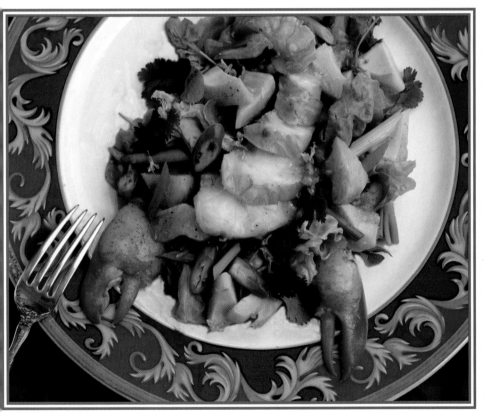

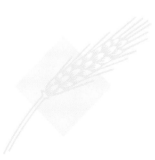

Shrimp Risotto with Red Onion and Corn

(see recipe on page 240)

Salad of Grapefruit, Orange, Fennel, and Field Greens

(see recipe on page 202)

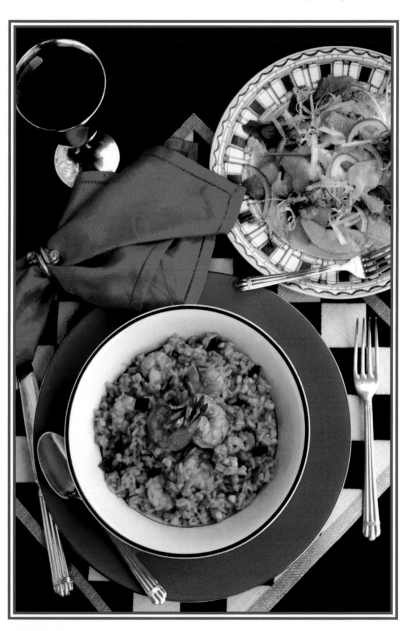

Spicy Chicken Soup

(see recipe on page 194)

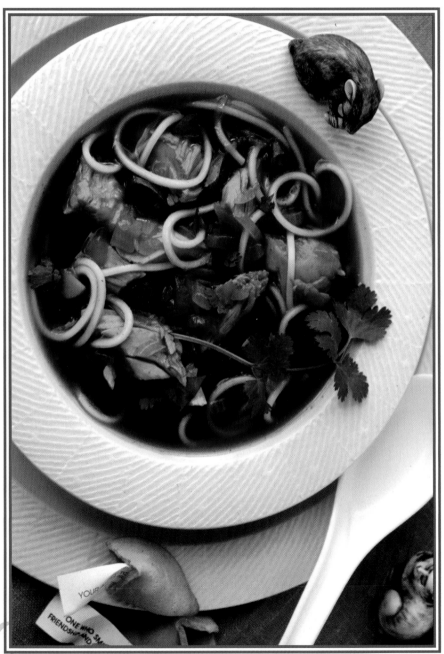

Duck Breasts Stuffed with Couscous Roasted with a Chermoula Coat and Served on a Lemon Lake

(see recipe on page 286)

Vegetable Couscous

(see recipe on page 228)

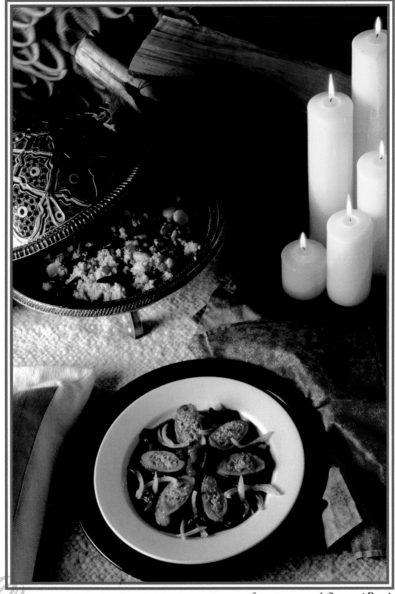

Setting courtesy of Crate and Barrel

ROASTED OSTRICH IN A CHIPOTLE MARINADE OVER CREAMY POLENTA

(see recipes on pages 294 and 230)

CORN-STUFFED CHILIES WITH STRAWBERRY PAPAYA SALSA

(see recipes on pages 216 and 160)

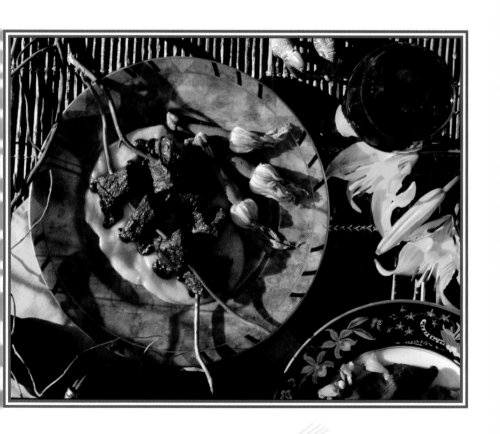

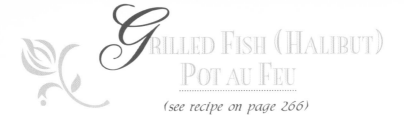

Grilled Fish (Halibut) Pot au Feu

(see recipe on page 266)

Green Salad with Pears and Persimmons

(add slices of pear and persimmon to your favorite green salad)

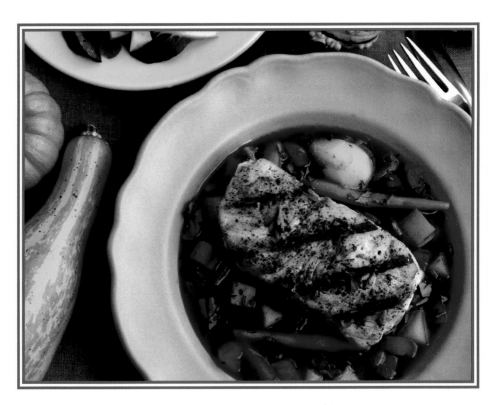

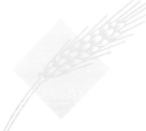

MEDITERRANEAN CHICKEN

(see recipe on page 276)

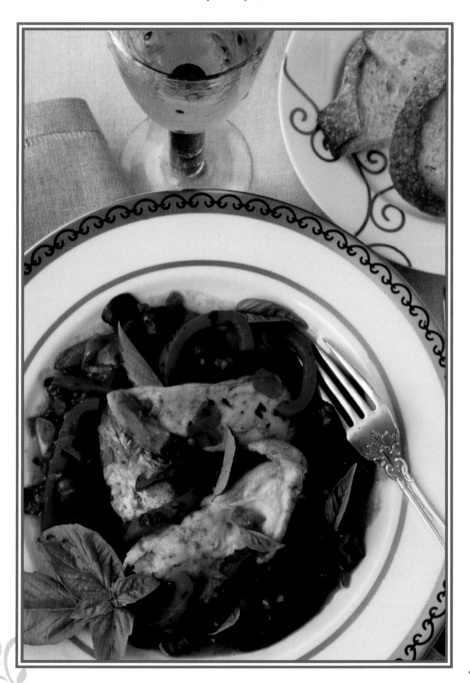

ROASTED RED SNAPPER WITH GRILLED TOMATILLO SALSA

(see recipe on page 260)

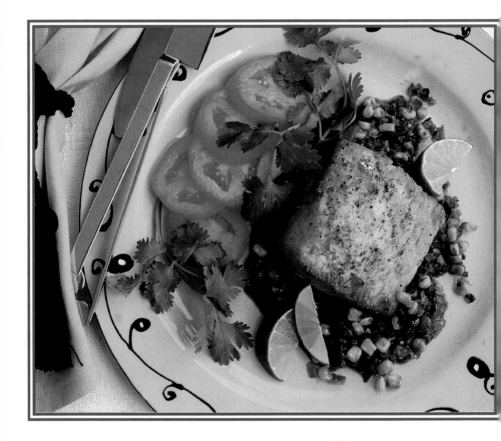

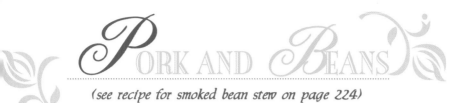

PORK AND BEANS

(see recipe for smoked bean stew on page 224)

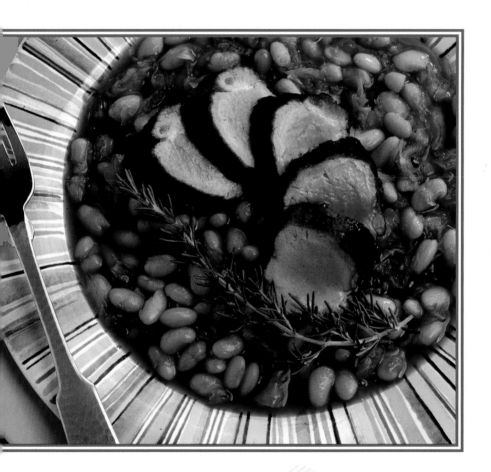

Strawberry Mango and Green Apple Sorbets on Meringue with Blueberry Sauce

(see recipes on pages 302 and 306)

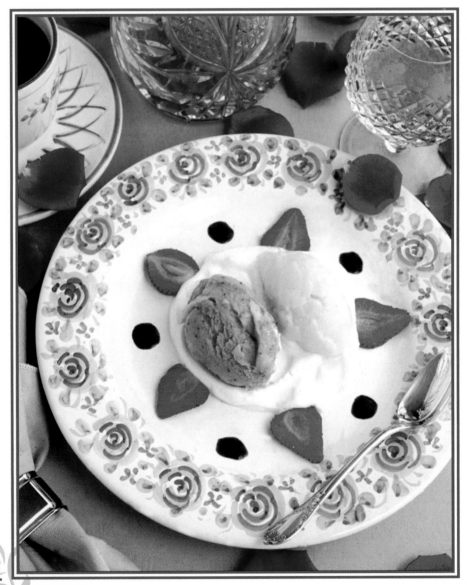

Appetizers
and
First Courses

MOC-GUAC (LOW-FAT GUACAMOLE)
Quick and Easy

78 calories per serving

Prep Time: 10 minutes
Cook Time: 6 minutes (peas)

> 2 cups peas, cooked and pureed
> $^1/_2$ onion, chopped fine
> 1 jalapeno chili,* chopped fine
> 1 tsp. ground cumin* (or cumin seeds)
> 2 Tbsp. cilantro,* chopped
> 2 Tbsp. vegetable oil
> $^1/_8$ cup lime or lemon juice
> $^1/_8$ tsp. cayenne pepper

––––––––––––––––––––––––––– ❧ –––––––––––––––––––––––––––

Combine all ingredients. Serve as a dip with vegetable sticks.

––––––––––––––––––––––––––– ❧ –––––––––––––––––––––––––––

Serves 8

We think this is one of the more fun recipes. Avocado is very high in saturated fat. This version tastes almost the same, but is very low in fat. Have your friends guess what the main ingredient is. Most of ours can't.

*Information on this ingredient is included in the Glossary.

Appetizers and First Courses

TRADITIONAL SALSA
Quick and Easy

14 calories per serving

Prep Time: 15 minutes
Cook Time: 0

> 1 to 2 tomatoes, chopped (1 cup chopped)
> 1/2 onion, chopped (1/2 cup chopped)
> 1 jalapeno chili,* chopped
> 4 Tbsp. cilantro,* chopped
> 1 Tbsp. lemon or lime juice
> 1/4 tsp. salt (or to taste)
> 1/8 tsp. pepper
> 1/8 tsp. sugar

———————————— ❦ ————————————

Combine all ingredients. Allow to rest for 30 minutes (or more) so that flavors will blend.

———————————— ❦ ————————————

Serves 6 as a dip

*Information on this ingredient is included in the Glossary.

STRAWBERRY PAPAYA SALSA

Quick and Easy

85 calories per serving

Prep Time: 10 minutes
Cook Time: 0

$^1/_2$ onion, diced
8 strawberries, diced
$^1/_2$ papaya, diced
4 Tbsp. parsley stems, diced
1 Tbsp. apple cider vinegar
1 serrano* or jalapeno chili* or less (to taste), chopped
juice of 1 orange
juice of 1 lime
$^1/_2$ tsp. salt
$^1/_8$ tsp. ground black pepper

———————————————— ❧ ————————————————

Combine all ingredients. Allow to rest at least 15 minutes before serving so that flavors will combine.

———————————————— ❧ ————————————————

Serves 6 as an hors d'oeuvre with raw vegetables

This dish makes a good accompaniment to spicy food such as stuffed chilies. The colors are so beautiful, this salsa dresses up any dish.

*Information on this ingredient is included in the Glossary.

Appetizers and First Courses

CUCUMBER DIP
Quick and Easy

54 calories per serving

Prep Time: 15 minutes
Cook Time: 0

1 cucumber, peeled and seeded
1 bunch green onions, green part only, coarsely chopped
lemon juice to taste
$^1/_2$ tsp. salt
$^1/_8$ to $^1/_4$ tsp. cayenne pepper
8 oz. nonfat cream cheese

Combine cucumber, onions, salt and pepper in a blender or food processor. Blend until well pureed and there is some liquid in the bottom of the blender. Add nonfat cream cheese and blend until well combined. Add lemon juice to taste and correct the seasonings if necessary. Chill at least one hour before serving. May be made a day ahead. Serve with fresh vegetables.

Serves about 6 as an hors d'oeuvre

HUMMUS
Quick and Easy

112 calories per serving

Prep Time: 10 minutes
Cook Time: 0

> 1 can (about 1½ cups) chick peas (garbanzo beans),
>   rinsed and drained
> ½ cup water
> ½ tsp. salt
> 2 cloves garlic, finely chopped
> ¼ tsp. black pepper
> ¼ tsp. sesame oil
> ¼ cup fresh lemon juice

———————————————— ❧ ————————————————

Combine all ingredients in a blender or food processor and blend until well pureed.

———————————————— ❧ ————————————————

Serves 8–10 as a dip

Hummus makes a good low-fat dip served with vegetable sticks or toasted pita triangles. It is also wonderful served as an accompaniment to tabbouleh (see recipe on page 207).

Appetizers and First Courses

CLAM COCKTAILS
Quick and Easy

34 calories per serving

Prep Time: 15 minutes
Cook Time: 0

> 12 live cherrystone clams = about 18 littleneck =
>   about 2+ lbs.
> 2 Tbsp. tomato, chopped
> 2 Tbsp. cilantro, chopped
> 2 Tbsp. red onion, chopped
> 2 jalapeno chilies,* chopped
> 2 Tbsp. catsup
> juice of 2 limes
> $1/4$ tsp. or less salt (to taste)

Remove clams from their shells. Save the liquid. Chop clams coarsely. Add clams and liquid to all the other ingredients. Salt to taste. Mix well. Refrigerate. Serve in clam shells with a cocktail fork, or serve in small shooter glasses. Makes about 24 shooters.

Serves 4–6

*Information on this ingredient is included in the Glossary.

SMOKED SCALLOPS AND SHRIMP

Quick and Easy

61 calories per serving

Prep Time: 5 minutes
Cook Time: 15 minutes

8 shrimps, shelled
8 scallops

Marinade:
1 tsp. oil
2 garlic cloves, chopped
1 Tbsp. parsley, chopped
$1/8$ tsp. black pepper
2 Tbsp. lemon juice
pinch of salt or to taste

hickory or mesquite wood chips for smoking, soaked in water

───────────── ❧ ─────────────

Mix the seafood with the marinade and set aside in the refrigerator for 30 to 60 minutes. Place soaked smoking chips (mesquite or hickory) in a cast-iron skillet or wok and cover with a grid. Then cover with a domed top and heat for 10 minutes (until smoking). Place scallops and shrimp on the grid and cover. Smoke for 10 minutes. Remove. Heat remaining marinade in a nonstick pan, and briefly saute shrimp and scallops on high heat.

Skewer and serve with your favorite sauce. Try the low-fat barbeque sauce (see recipe on page 315) with this dish.

───────────── ❧ ─────────────

Serves 4 as an appetizer

Try this as a tasty alternative to beef barbeque!

BROILED CLAMS WITH MISO AND SAKE

Quick and Adventurous

164 calories per serving

Prep Time: 20 minutes
Cook Time: 5–7 minutes

20 littleneck clams (cherrystones are okay, too)
2 Tbsp. red miso*
2 Tbsp. rice wine vinegar
2 Tbsp. sake
4 tsp. chili oil
2 tsp. sesame oil
pinch pepper
chopped chives

———————————————— ❦ ————————————————

Shuck the clams and place them back into their shells, SAVING THE JUICE. Strain the juice (you will have about $^1/_2$ cup). Combine the juice with all of the other ingredients and mix well. Spoon over clams. Place under broiler until they begin to bubble. Remove and serve immediately.

———————————————— ❦ ————————————————

Serves 4 as an appetizer or first course

*Information on this ingredient is included in the Glossary.

OYSTERS JULIA WITH DASHI

Quick and Adventurous

232 calories per serving

Prep Time: 20 minutes
Cook Time: 5 minutes

Dashi:
1 oz. dried seaweed*
15 grams bonito flakes*
4 cups water

Oysters:
5 large Pacific oysters, roughly
   chopped (save all the liquid!)
1 Tbsp. ginger puree
2 tsp. soy sauce
2 tsp. rice vinegar
5 drops chili oil
5 drops sesame oil

6 Napa cabbage leaves,
   steamed
1 bulb fennel, julienned
2 ribs celery, julienned
1 carrot, julienned

———————————— ❧ ————————————

Steam the Napa cabbage leaves and save. Combine the oysters, ginger puree, soy, rice vinegar, chili, and sesame oils in a bowl and mix well. Make the dashi; place the seaweed and water in a pot and bring to a boil. After simmering for 5 minutes, add the bonito flakes and turn off the heat. Let the mixture infuse for 5–10 minutes and then strain, discarding the solids.

Add oyster liquid to the dashi. Divide the oyster mixture and spoon onto the Napa cabbage. Fold up the cabbage enclosing the oysters. Place in a steamer and steam for 5 minutes. Meanwhile, add the vegetables (fennel, celery, carrot) to the dashi, and simmer while you're awaiting the oysters.

Place cabbage rolls two to a plate (or one, depending on use), and spoon over the dashi with the veggies.

———————————— ❧ ————————————

Serves 3 with two packs each, or 6 people with one roll

*Information on this ingredient is included in the Glossary.

SEAFOOD PACKS
Quick and Easy

65 calories per serving

Prep Time: 10 minutes
Cook Time: 5 minutes

12 iceberg lettuce leaves
1 doz. oysters, shucked (save the liquid)
$1/2$ lb. scallops
1 tsp. tarragon, chopped
1 dry red chili, crumbled
1 Tbsp. Pernod
salt to taste
$1/8$ tsp. ground black pepper

2 cups homemade nonfat vegetable or fish stock
  (see recipes on pages 130-131)

Steam the lettuce leaves for 2 minutes, or until they are pliable. Chop the oysters and scallops. Mix with the other ingredients. Place a small amount (about one heaping Tbsp.) on each lettuce leaf and wrap by folding like an envelope so that the mixture is totally encased. Steam over broth (vegetable or fish) for 2 minutes and serve.

Serves 6

SHRIMP TIMBALES
Quick and Easy

216 calories per serving

Prep Time: 10 minutes
Cook Time: 25 minutes

> 1 lb. shrimp, shelled
> 4 egg whites
> 4 green onions, chopped
> 1 stalk celery, chopped
> 1 carrot, chopped
> 2 Tbsp. chervil,* chopped
> 4 tsp. lemon juice
> $1/8$ tsp. ground pepper
> 4 tsp. water
> 2 tsp. peanut oil

❧

Beat the egg whites. Put the shrimp in a blender or food processor, and puree. Heat the oil. Saute the green onions, celery, carrot, and chervil until tender. Cool. Add lemon juice. Combine with the shrimp and egg whites. Add salt and pepper to taste. Mix well. Spray 4 ramekins* (3-$1/2$"–4" in diameter) with a vegetable spray such as PAM. Spoon mixture into ramekins, and bake in a 350-degree oven in a pan of hot water for 15 minutes. Unmold by running a knife along the edge of each ramekin, and turn upside down on a plate.

❧

Serves 4

This low-fat dish is great with a simple salad of watercress dressed with a light vinaigrette.

*Information on this term or ingredient is included in the Glossary.

CRAB WONTONS

Appetizers and First Courses

Adventurous

272 calories per serving

Prep Time: 20 minutes
Cook Time: 15 minutes

wonton skins
1 tsp. mustard oil

Filling:
$^1/_3$ lb. crab meat (5.5 oz.)
2 oz. lean ground pork (from tenderloin)
3 green onions, green part only, chopped
1 clove garlic, minced
3 Tbsp. watercress, chopped
5 water chestnuts, chopped (3 Tbsp.)
4 tsp. rice vinegar
$^1/_2$ tsp. soy sauce
$^1/_2$ tsp. sesame oil
1 tsp. chili oil
1 tsp. ginger paste (or 1 Tbsp. grated fresh ginger)
3 tsp. lemon juice

Combine the filling ingredients.

Place a small amount of filling in the middle of a wonton skin. Wet the edges of the wonton with a little water and fold over to make a triangle. Boil the wontons gently for 2 minutes. Then fry in a nonstick pan in one teaspoon mustard oil until brown.

Serve with your favorite Chinese sauce (for example, plum or chili) or, for a fun twist, try them with adobo sauce (see recipe on page 288).

Makes 24
Serves 6

BANGKOK BURRITOS WITH HOT THAI PEANUT SAUCE

Adventurous

100 calories per serving

Prep Time: 20 minutes
Cook Time: 7 minutes

      rice paper
      water

Burritos:
4 oz. (280 gm.) minced chicken
4 oz. (280 gm.) minced shrimp
4 oz. (280 gm.) bean sprouts
1 Tbsp. lime juice
1 Tbsp. hot Thai sauce (see next page)
2 green onions, sliced on diagonal.
1 Tbsp. ginger, chopped
4 oz. cabbage, chopped
1 carrot, peeled and coarsely grated
6 rice paper sheets
fish sauce to taste
pepper to taste

Mix the burrito ingredients. Check for seasoning, and correct with fish sauce and pepper as needed. Place a rice paper in water, and allow to soften (but not too much!). Drain and put on a clean surface. Spoon 3–4 tablespoons of mixture onto one side of the paper. Roll up as if you were wrapping a gift package. Place loose end down in a steamer. Repeat until you have used all of the burrito filling. This amount should make 8–10 burritos that are about 5" x 1.5" x 1".

BANGKOK BURRITOS (CONT.)

Prepare the hot Thai sauce by combining:
>   5 small garlic cloves, sliced
>   2 small garlic cloves, crushed
>   2 chili chipotles*, finely minced
> $1/2$ cup lemon juice
> $1/4$ cup fish sauce* or less
>   3 Tbsp. cilantro*, finely chopped
>   1 Tbsp. sugar or maple syrup

To prepare the hot Thai peanut sauce, combine:
> $1/2$ cup peanut butter
>   1 cup hot Thai sauce
> $1/2$ cup water

Steam the burritos for about 5–7 minutes. Place on a plate with sauce, and serve.

Serves 4–6

*Information on this ingredient is included in the Glossary.

SALMON TARTARE
Quick and Adventurous

73 calories per serving

Prep Time: 10 minutes
Cook Time: 0

Per Serving:
3 oz. fresh salmon fillet, skin removed
1 tsp. capers
1 tsp. horseradish
1 tsp. Dijon mustard
1 heaping tsp. green onions, chopped
1 heaping tsp. red onions, chopped

Optional:
1 raw quail egg*
1 tsp. flying fish eggs*
uni*

Grind the salmon in a meat grinder, or chop it if you have no grinder. Place a mound of salmon in the middle of the plate. Surround the salmon with little mounds of the condiments. If you use a quail egg, make an indentation in the middle of the salmon, remove from shell, and separate out the yolk. Place the yolk on the salmon. Sprinkle the dish with flying fish eggs.
Serve with toast points (thin bread cut into triangles and toasted).

Serves one

This is one of the most popular dishes we serve as a first course. Even people who don't like sushi like this. It is EASY, QUICK, and DELICIOUS.

*Information on this ingredient is included in the Glossary.

Appetizers and First Courses

GRAVLACHS
Quick and Easy

197 calories per serving

Prep Time: 15 minutes
Cook Time: 0 minutes (or 3 days, depending on how you look at it)

      1 side of salmon (2–3 lbs.), boned, skin on
      1 bunch tarragon
      1 bunch basil
      1 bunch dill
      1 bunch parsley
      1 bunch thyme
      1 shallot, chopped
      3 green onions, chopped
      $^1/_3$ cup salt
      1 cup sugar

Chop the herbs together with the shallots and onions. Mix well. Place the salmon on a baking pan lined with plastic wrap flesh side up. Cover with the herb mixture. Mix salt and sugar and sprinkle on top of herbs and onions. Cover with plastic wrap. Add a heavy weight on top. Place in the refrigerator and let it "cook" for three days. Remove from the refrigerator, and scrape off the herbs and seasonings (I wash the fillet under cold running water). Drain.

Slice very thinly, and serve with toast points or toasted crackers.

Serves 10–12

This recipe requires room in your refrigerator. It is important to weigh the fish down with a heavy weight. We use a case of wine or mineral water. Barbells or a pail of water will also work. Even though the recipe includes substantial salt, the amount of salt that actually gets into the fish is minuscule. It will not taste at all salty, but will be infused with the fragrance of the herbs.

CHICKEN TIKKA DRUMETTES
Quick and Adventurous

200 calories per serving

Prep Time: 5 minutes
Cook Time: 15 minutes

16 chicken drumettes

2 Tbsp. kebab spice paste*
2 Tbsp. tikka paste*
2 Tbsp. mustard oil*
3 cloves garlic, chopped
2 Tbsp. lemon juice.

―――――――――――――――― ❧ ――――――――――――――――

Combine all of the tikka ingredients, and mix well before you put drumettes into the mixture. Mix well again, and place in the refrigerator for 30 minutes to 24 hours.

When you are ready to cook, bring the meat to room temperature and grill.

―――――――――――――――― ❧ ――――――――――――――――

Makes appetizers for 4

*Information on this ingredient is included in the Glossary.

LARB

Quick and Adventurous

200 calories per serving

Prep Time: 15 minutes
Cook Time: 7 minutes

1 lb. chicken breast, ground or minced
3 green onions, sliced thin
$^1/_4$ cup red onion, sliced paper thin
4 pieces galanga* (optional, but makes the dish even better)
3 Tbsp. fish sauce*
$^1/_4$ cup homemade nonfat chicken stock (see recipe on page 132)
    or canned nonfat broth
$^1/_4$ cup lime juice
$1^1/_2$ tsp. ground roasted red chilies (this may be too spicy for you;
    try adding $^1/_2$ tsp. at a time to your taste)
2 Tbsp. ground toasted rice
1 shallot, sliced thin
$^1/_2$ stalk lemon grass* (if you can get it), finely chopped
finely sliced romaine leaves

—————————————— ❧ ——————————————

Heat a nonstick skillet or wok, and toast the uncooked rice (without oil), stirring constantly, until lightly brown. It will take 3–4 minutes. Remove and grind in a blender or coffee grinder. Roast the chilies in the hot dry skillet until blackened, then grind and set aside. Brown the galanga in the same pan. Grind and set aside. Now add the chicken to the dry pan and stir-fry quickly until the meat is white and cooked through. In a pan, heat the fish sauce, chicken broth, and lime juice. Add the green onion, red onion, shallot, and lemon grass. Turn off the heat and toss in the chilies (to taste), galanga, rice, and chicken. Combine and serve.

—————————————— ❧ ——————————————

Serves 4–6

Serve on a platter surrounded by romaine leaves. This wonderful Thai dish is traditionally served by spooning the chicken mixture on the romaine leaves and eating by hand. The toasted rice can be made ahead and kept in a jar indefinitely. Larb can be a main-course salad for lunch (serves 3), an hors d'oeuvre, or an accompaniment to a meal. Delicious!

*Information on this ingredient is included in the Glossary.

STUFFED GRAPE LEAVES

Adventurous

52 calories per serving

Prep Time: 40 minutes
Cook Time: 40 minutes

> 30 large or 60 small grape leaves (8 oz. jar)
> 2 onions, chopped fine (3 cups chopped)
> 1 tsp. olive oil
> $3/4$ cup uncooked long grain rice (Basmati is best)
> 2 Tbsp. mint, chopped fine
> 2 Tbsp. parsley, chopped fine
> 2 tomatoes, peeled, seeded, and chopped
> $1/2$ tsp. ground allspice
> $1/2$ tsp. ground cumin*
> $1/2$ tsp. salt
> $1/2$ tsp. pepper
> $1/2$ cup raisins, plumped (by boiling in 1 cup water for 3 minutes)
> 2 Tbsp. lemon juice
> 1 cup homemade nonfat chicken or vegetable stock (see recipes on
>   pages 131–132), or canned nonfat broth
> water

Rinse the grape leaves, then blanch in simmering water for 5 minutes. Rinse in cold water. Heat the oil in a nonstick pan and saute the onions until soft, about 10 minutes. In a bowl, combine all ingredients except the grape leaves and broth. Put a spoonful of the mixture in the middle of each grape leaf. Fold up the sides of the leaf to cover the rice mixture, then roll up the leaf. In a saucepan, place stuffed leaves very close to each other so that they won't unfold while cooking. Cover the leaves with broth and enough water to just cover the leaves. Simmer, covered, for 30–40 minutes or until rice inside leaves is cooked.

Serves 12–16 as an appetizer, or 8 as a main course

These dolmas can be made very small, about 1" x 2" with small leaves as an appetizer, or about 2" x 4" as a main-course dish with larger leaves. If you want to make small ones, but only have large leaves, try using $1/2$ leaf for each, or trim the leaves with scissors. The larger ones take a little longer to cook.

*Information on this ingredient is included in the Glossary.

SHIITAKE OPEN-FACED SANDWICHES
Quick and Adventurous

204 calories per serving

Prep Time: 25 minutes
Cook Time: 10 minutes

> 24 fresh shiitake mushrooms*
> 1 lb. sea scallops
> 3–4 sea urchin ovaries (uni*) or 1 Tbsp. processed
> 2 tsp. Aji-pon sauce*

Dashi:
3" Konbu (dried seaweed)
1 oz. finely shredded dried bonito flakes*
4–5 cups water
2 tsp. cornstarch dissolved in 2 Tbsp. water
2 tsp. white miso*
1 tsp. soy sauce

1–2 yamagobo root, finely diced*
2 green onions, green part only, finely sliced

Make the Dashi: Combine the water and the konbu, and heat to boiling. Add the bonito, and stir and remove from the heat. Let the pot come to room temperature. Strain, keeping the liquid (the solids can be used for "second" dashi). Use one cup dashi, and add the white miso and the soy. Heat and add the cornstarch. Bring this mixture to a boil and immediately take it off the flame. If it is too thick, add some water. If it's not thick enough, add a little more cornstarch. (The sauce should be more "runny" than clotted.) Keep warm.

Puree the scallops and sea urchin. Add the Aji-pon. Mix well. Fill the underside of the shiitake mushrooms with a teaspoon or more (depending on the size of the mushroom) of the scallop mixture. Heat a nonstick pan, sprayed first with a vegetable oil, and place the mushrooms CAP DOWN in the hot pan. Let them cook for 2–3 minutes, then turn them over to quickly cook the other side.

Ladle some of the dashi onto plates to cover the bottom evenly. Place 6 mushrooms, cap up, in a circle in the middle of each plate. Sprinkle some yamagobo in the center, and the green onions around the perimeter. Serve immediately.

Serves 4

*Information on this ingredient may be found in the Glossary.

RAVIOLI WITHOUT RAVIOLI

Adventurous

374 calories per serving

Prep Time: 30 minutes
Cook Time: 20 minutes

1 large turnip, peeled

Filling:
5 shiitake mushrooms,* chopped
$^1/_4$ cup wood ear mushrooms,* chopped
2 green onions, green part only, chopped
2 tsp. mushroom soy sauce*
$^1/_4$ tsp. sesame oil
6 oz. red wine
6 oz. homemade nonfat chicken or vegetable stock
    (see recipes on pages 131–132), or canned nonfat broth
1 egg white, beaten until foamy

Sauce:
1 Tbsp. Mirin*
2 Tbsp. rice vinegar
1 shallot, chopped
1 inch ginger, peeled and chopped
12 oz. homemade nonfat chicken or vegetable broth
    (see recipes on pages 131–132), or canned nonfat broth
6 oz. nonfat plain yogurt

$^1/_2$ cup peanut oil
2 Tbsp. cilantro,* chopped

*Information on this ingredient is included in the Glossary.

RAVIOLI WITHOUT RAVIOLI (CONT.)

───────────────────── ❧ ─────────────────────

Prepare the filling. Combine all of the filling ingredients in a blender, except the egg white. After the ingredients are well pureed, add the egg white, folding it into the mixture with a spatula.

The sauce: Heat the Mirin, rice vinegar, shallot, and ginger in a pan. Add stock and reduce slowly, until slightly thickened. Add yogurt and stir until well blended. Strain and keep warm.

Assembly: Slice the turnip into half-inch discs. You should be able to get 4–6 slices. Parboil, steam, or microwave the slices for 3–5 minutes until pliable and slightly soft. When they are cooked, use a sharp knife and make a pocket in each turnip slice. Place the filling mixture in a pastry bag, and pipe some of the mixture into each turnip pocket. Do not overfill.

Cook: Heat the oil in the wok until smoke begins to rise. Drop in a ravioli turnip. Cook until golden. Drain on paper towels.

To serve: Place some sauce on each plate, and put a ravioli in the middle of the plate. Sprinkle with cilantro.

───────────────────── ❧ ─────────────────────

Serves 4

DAIKON RADISH SANDWICH ON ASIAN NOODLES AND CARROT JUS

Adventurous

211 calories per serving

Prep Time: 30 minutes
Cook Time: 10 minutes

1 daikon radish*
1 cup frozen mixed veggies, chopped
1 shallot, chopped
8 snow peas
$^1/_8$ tsp. salt and pepper, mixed

Noodle:
8 oz. of yam noodles* (almost 0 calories) or glass
   noodles, or rice sticks (soaked in water until soft)

Carrot Jus:
10 carrots
$^1/_2$ tsp. lemon juice
water

Slice daikon radish $^1/_{16}$" thick or as thin as possible. Steam or poach slices until pliable, about 2 minutes. Bring water to boil in a steamer. Spray steaming rack with vegetable spray. Combine veggie mixture and spread on radish slices. Top each with another slice and place in steamer insert. Cover and steam about 4 minutes, or until radish is transparent and you can see the colors of the vegetable through the radish.

*Information on this ingredient is included in the Glossary.

Appetizers and First Courses

DAIKON RADISH SANDWICH (CONT.)

Cook the carrots until very tender. Puree and cook over low heat until VERY thick. The carrots will caramelize, and their natural sweetness will come through. Stir frequently to avoid burning. After thickening, add lemon juice and enough water to make 6 tablespoons.

Rinse and strain noodles, and toss with carrot jus.

To serve, place a nest of the noodle and carrot jus mixture on each plate. Top with steamed daikon sandwiches. Decorate with steamed snow peas.

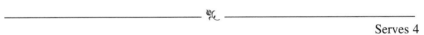

Serves 4

This is a little unusual and really good.

First-Course
and
Main-Dish Soups

CREAMED CORN SOUP
(WITHOUT CREAM!)
Quick and Easy

94 calories per servng

Prep Time: 15 minutes
Cook Time: 30 minutes

^{1}/2 red onion, chopped
1 shallot, chopped
1 pasilla chili,* peeled and chopped
1 Tbsp. corn oil
kernels from 3 ears of corn
2 cups homemade chicken stock
  (see recipe on page 132) or canned nonfat broth
1^1/4 cups water
1^1/2 Tbsp. lemon juice
1 tsp. salt (or to taste)
pinch of sugar
2 Tbsp. cilantro,* chopped

Saute ^{1}/4 onion, shallot, and ^{1}/2 pasilla chili in corn oil for 3–4 minutes. Add the corn and stock and simmer for about 4 minutes, stirring frequently. Puree the mixture, then return it to the pot. Add the water and simmer 10 minutes, stirring occasionally. Add the rest of the onion and chili, the lemon juice, salt, and sugar, and simmer another 10 minutes. Serve hot with cilantro and a grind of pepper on top of each bowl.

Serves 4 (depending on size of bowl). Makes about 40 oz.

*Information on this ingredient is included in the Glossary. If you can't get a pasilla chili, substitute a green bell pepper or use ^{1}/4 tsp. black pepper.

First-Course and Main-Dish Soups

PUMPKIN SOUP
Quick and Easy

71 calories per serving

Prep Time: 20 minutes
Cook Time: 20 minutes

1 Tbsp. vegetable oil
1 onion, chopped
$^1/_2$ cup green onions, white part only, chopped
1 17-oz. can pumpkin (2 cups)
4 cups homemade nonfat chicken or vegetable stock (see
    recipes on pages 131–132) or canned nonfat broth
1 bay leaf
1 tsp. sugar
2 Tbsp. parsley, chopped
$^1/_4$ tsp. ground nutmeg
$^1/_4$ tsp. ground cinnamon
$1^1/_2$ cups nonfat milk or nonfat soy milk
2 Tbsp. lemon juice
salt and pepper to taste

Garnish: chopped chives and a spoon of fat-free yogurt
    or fat-free sour cream.

———————————— ❧ ————————————

Heat the oil in a nonstick pan. Slowly saute onion and green onions until soft and golden.

In the meantime, combine the pumpkin, stock, bay leaf, sugar, and parsley in a saucepan. When the onions are soft, add them to the other ingredients and simmer, covered, for 15 minutes. Remove the bay leaf, and stir in the nutmeg and cinnamon. Puree the soup in a blender or food processor until smooth. Return to the saucepan, and add milk and lemon juice. Heat through but do not boil. Add salt and pepper to taste.

———————————— ❧ ————————————

Serves 8

This is a great fall and winter dish. It's delicious served hot or cold, and it's even better if you make it a day or two before you serve it.

"TWO CUP" MUSHROOM BARLEY SOUP
Quick and Easy

258 calories per serving

Prep Time: 10 minutes
Cook Time: 20 minutes

1 tsp. oil
2 cups celery (about 6 ribs), chopped
2 cups carrots (about 4 carrots), chopped
2 cups onion (about 1 big onion), chopped
2 cups portobello mushrooms*,
   (about 2 mushrooms), chopped
2 cups pearl barley
2 cups white wine
12 cups water
3 cloves garlic, chopped
2 tsp. salt
pinch pepper
1 tsp. dried thyme or 2 tsp. fresh thyme
1 Tbsp. tomato paste (optional)

———————————— ❧ ————————————

Put oil in a large pot. Saute the celery, carrots, onion, and garlic until they are dark tan. Add the pearl barley and mix well. Let the barley color slightly. Add the wine and water, salt, pepper, thyme, mushrooms (and tomato paste, if you wish). Simmer and skim off all of the oil as it rises to the surface. Cook gently until the barley is soft. Tomato paste is optional and, if desired, should be stirred in at this time until well distributed. Correct the seasonings and serve hot.

———————————— ❧ ————————————

Serves 8

*Information on this ingredient is included in the Glossary.

DARK YELLOW SQUASH SOUP

Easy

125 calories per serving

Prep Time: 10 minutes
Cook Time: 1 hour

2 large dark yellow squash (acorn, butternut, table
    queen, or other winter squash)
2 tsp. walnut oil
1 onion, finely chopped
"heat"
5 cups homemade nonfat chicken or vegetable stock (see
    recipes on pages 131–132) or canned nonfat broth
1 shallot, chopped
1 Tbsp. balsamic vinegar
$^1/_4$ tsp. salt, or to taste
2 cups water
$^1/_4$ cup rice wine vinegar*
chives or green onions, chopped
salt to taste

Take the squash and slice it in half. Wrap each piece in foil and place cut side down on a pan in a 350-degree (moderate) oven for 45 minutes. When the flesh feels soft through the foil, it's ready. Scrape out the seeds, and discard or plant. Scoop out flesh with a spoon or other suitable object. You should have about 2 cups. Mash it with a fork, or puree. In a skillet, heat the oil and saute the onion, "heat," and shallot until slightly brown. Add the squash puree and the balsamic vinegar. If the soup is too thick, add some water (up to 2 cups) depending on the thickness of the puree. Heat to a simmer so that the ingredients can blend thoroughly. Add the rice wine vinegar, and heat through. Serve in a bowl garnished with chopped chives or green onions.

Serves 6

*Information on this ingredient is included in the Glossary.

BROCCOLI SOUP
Quick and Easy

173 calories per serving

Prep Time: 15 minutes
Cook Time: 15 minutes

> 4 cups broccoli, about one pound, steamed
> 1 medium onion, chopped
> 3 cloves garlic, chopped
> "heat"
> 1 tsp. walnut oil
> $1/2$ tsp. salt
> 1 Tbsp. lemon juice
> pinch sugar
> 4 cups homemade nonfat chicken stock (see recipe on
>   page 132) or canned nonfat broth
> parsley for garnish

———————————————— ❧ ————————————————

Clean the broccoli and steam until tender. Puree in a blender with some stock or broth or water. In a nonstick pan, roast the onion and garlic in one teaspoon walnut oil until brown. Place the onion and garlic in a soup pot, and add the broccoli puree, the stock or broth, salt, lemon juice, "heat," and sugar. Bring to a simmer, and add more liquid if too thick. Correct the seasonings, and serve hot with a sprinkle of parsley on top.

———————————————— ❧ ————————————————

Serves 2–4

GAZPACHO
Adventurous

49 calories per serving

Prep Time: 40 minutes
Cook Time: 0

2 cups homemade nonfat chicken or vegetable stock
(see recipes on pages 131–132) or canned nonfat broth
2 cups V-8 or any vegetable juice
1 cucumber, peeled and seeded (or $2/3$ of a hothouse cucumber)

Puree and strain the cucumber and blend with the broth and
vegetable juice in a large bowl.

Combine the following ingredients with the liquid:
1 Tbsp. red wine vinegar
$1/2$ red onion, chopped (about 1 cup)
$1/2$ cucumber (or $1/3$ hothouse cucumber), seeded and finely diced
1 firm tomato, seeded and finely diced (1 heaping cup)
1 clove garlic, chopped fine
1 stalk celery, chopped fine
1 jalapeno chili,* chopped fine
$1/2$ red or green bell pepper, finely diced
2 Tbsp. chopped parsley
1 tsp. salt
$1/8$ tsp. pepper
2 Tbsp. lemon juice
2 dashes cayenne pepper (or to taste)
$1/4$ tsp. cumin seed or ground cumin*

To serve: Chill for at least 2 hours to allow the flavors to blend.
Ladle into bowls. Add a squeeze of lemon and serve.

Optional: If you'd like a change, try blending in one cup fat-free
yogurt for a Creamed Gazpacho.

Serves 6

*Information on this ingredient is included in the Glossary.

BLACK BEAN SOUP

Adventurous

254 calories per serving

Prep Time: 20 minutes
Cook Time: 1^1/$_2$ hours

1 lb. black beans, soaked
   in enough water to cover them
1^1/$_2$ onions, chopped
5 cloves garlic, chopped
1 smoked ham hock (about 3 oz.)
1 Tbsp. vegetable oil
8 cups water
2 bay leaves
4 cloves
1 tsp. cumin seeds*
1 pasilla chili,* skinned
   and seeded (optional)

1 bunch cilantro,* chopped
1 tsp. dry oregano
^{1}/$_3$ cup apple cider vinegar
2 Tbsp. fresh oregano
1 tsp. salt
1 Tbsp. lemon juice
^{1}/$_2$ tsp. ground black pepper
1 cup tomato, chopped (optional)
1 chipotle chili* (optional)

    Heat the oil in a deep pot. Add the onions, garlic, and ham hock, and saute until onions are transparent. (Don't worry about the fat on the ham hock. We'll take it out later after the flavor gets in.) Rinse the beans and add to the pot. Stir. Add the water, bay leaves, cloves, cumin seeds, and pasilla chili. Bring to a low boil. Skim off the foam and any fat that rises to the top. Add half the cilantro and the dry oregano. Cook on low heat, covered, for 30 minutes. Skim off any foam or fat that rises to the top. Remove the ham hock. Take the meat off the bone. Remove any fat. Chop the meat and add it back to the soup. Cover and simmer for 30 minutes more.

    Take out 1^1/$_2$ cups beans, and puree. Add back to soup with vinegar, fresh oregano, salt, tomatoes, and chipotle chili. Cook until flavors are well combined and beans are cooked (10–30 minutes). Add lemon juice, the other half of the cilantro, and black pepper, and serve.

Serves 6–8

*Information on this ingredient is included in the Glossary.

First-Course and Main-Dish Soups

SMOKED SHRIMP AND TOMATO SOUP
Adventurous

190 calories per serving

Prep Time: 20 minutes
Cook Time: 20 minutes

> 13 Roma tomatoes or 4 cups tomato purée
> 1 onion, chopped
> 2 cloves garlic, chopped
> "heat"
> 10 cups homemade chicken stock
>   (see recipe on page 132) or canned nonfat broth
> lemon juice
> pinch sugar
> $1/2$ lb. shrimp, peeled (save the shells)
> 1 Tbsp. parsley, chopped

Peel the shrimp and save the shells. Peel and seed the tomatoes. Puree the tomatoes in a blender. You will have about 4 cups. In a stockpot, heat some oil and saute the onions, garlic, and "heat." Smoke the shrimp shells in a smoker for 10 minutes. Add the shells to the onions, etc., and add 4 cups broth. Simmer for 10 minutes and strain. Keep the liquid, and add the tomato puree, the sugar, and the rest (6 cups) of the broth. Simmer, skimming and cleaning the surface. Take a few of the shrimp and grind or mince them. Add to the soup and stir to disperse. Slice the other shrimp. Add all the shrimp, lemon juice to taste, and correct the seasonings. Simmer until shrimp are cooked. Serve in bowls with sprinkled parsley.

Serves 4

First-Course and Main-Dish Soups

LOBSTER SOUP WITH ARTICHOKES

Adventurous

166 calories per serving

Prep Time: 30 minutes
Cook Time: 20 minutes

3 shallots, chopped	$1/16$ tsp. ground saffron*
2 artichokes	lemon juice
1 lobster	1 cup white wine
1 tsp. oil	2 cups lobster broth (see below)
1 sprig thyme	1 Tbsp. Pernod
1 cup tomato puree	water
2 Tbsp. parsley, chopped	salt and pepper to taste

Steam the artichokes. Take off the leaves, remove and discard the choke, and cut the heart into half-inch cubes. Scrape the flesh off the leaves into a bowl and puree with 1–2 tablespoons water, then strain by pushing through a sieve. You will have about $3/4$ cup of artichoke puree.

Steam the lobster. Then remove the flesh from the shell and save. Chop shells, add the runny parts of the inside of the lobster to them and 4 cups of water. Simmer for 15 minutes while you are preparing the artichokes. This is the lobster broth.

In a nonstick pan, add one teaspoon oil and gently saute the 2 chopped shallots. Pour off all of the oil, and add the artichoke puree, the thyme, one cup white wine, and 2 cups of the lobster broth. Simmer for a few minutes. Add the tomato puree and simmer for 15 minutes, at least until the tomatoes are cooked and everything is nicely combined. Add broth to make a more soupy consistency (you should have about 4 cups) and taste for seasoning. Add salt, pepper, and/or lemon juice as necessary. Add one tablespoon Pernod and the saffron, and bubble for 3–4 minutes. Taste for and correct seasoning again.

Ladle the soup (one cup per serving) into a bowl, add the artichoke cubes and the lobster meat in a decorative way, and sprinkle on one tablespoon raw minced shallots and 2 tablespoons chopped parsley. Serve.

Serves 4; can be stretched to 6

*Information on this ingredient is included in the Glossary.

BOUILLABAISSE
Easy

475 calories per serving

Prep Time: 15 minutes
Cook Time: 15 minutes

> 10 shrimp, peeled
> 2 lbs. clams, scrubbed
> 1 lb. cockles*
> $^1/3$ lb. tuna, cubed
> $^1/3$ lb. escolar,* cubed (or other white fish)
> 1 lobster, steamed, meat removed and cubed
> 2 leeks, julienned
> grated rind of 2 oranges
> 4 tomatoes, peeled, seeded, and chopped
> 8 cups stock or broth (can be vegetable, fish, or poultry)
> a pinch saffron*
> 2 Tbsp. Pernod
> thyme
> oregano
> salt
> "heat"
> olive oil

Place shrimp, tuna, escolar, and lobster in a bowl with a generous pinch of thyme, oregano, salt, and "heat," plus one tablespoon olive oil. Mix well and set aside. In a large pot, saute the leeks in a tiny bit of oil. Add the stock, saffron, Pernod, tomatoes, and orange rind. Let this cook for 10 minutes (or more, if possible) at low heat to combine the ingredients. Skim. Add the shrimp, clams, and cockles. Simmer for 3–4 minutes and then add the fish and lobster. Skim. Bring to a boil, skim, lower heat, and serve hot.

Serves 4–6

*Information on this ingredient is included in the Glossary.

First-Course and Main-Dish Soups

SPICY CHICKEN SOUP

Adventurous

298 calories per serving

Prep Time: 30 minutes
Cook Time: 45 minutes

1 chicken, cut up
8 cups homemade nonfat chicken stock
   (see recipe on page 132) or canned nonfat broth
6 cups water
$1/4$ tsp. whole black peppercorns
1 onion, sliced
2 hot chilies (optional), sliced thin
1 Tbsp. peanut oil
1 Tbsp. curry powder
2 cloves garlic, chopped
$1^1/2$ tsp. ginger, chopped
1 tsp. shrimp paste*
1 tsp. ground turmeric*
1 tsp. ground coriander*
1 tsp. ground cumin*
$3^1/2$ oz. rice noodles (about half of most packages)
4 green onions, slivered
juice of 1 lemon
salt and pepper to taste
4 Tbsp. fresh cilantro,* chopped

Heat the chicken broth and water. Add the peppercorns, half an onion, and chicken. Simmer for 30 minutes. Skim off the fat, scum, and foam that rises to the top while cooking.

While the chicken is cooking, heat the oil in a nonstick pan, and saute

SPICY CHICKEN SOUP (CONT.)

the curry powder and the rest of the onion for three minutes. Add the garlic, chili, ginger, and shrimp paste, and stir over medium heat for 2 minutes. Add the turmeric, coriander, and cumin, and continue stirring for another minute.

When the chicken has finished cooking, strain the stock into a bowl. Remove the skin and bones from the chicken meat. Cut the meat into bite-size pieces and set aside. Put the stock back into its cooking pot, and add the cooked spices and onion. Simmer 10 minutes.

While the soup is simmering, soak the rice noodles in hot water for 10 minutes. Drain and cut into short (6") lengths. Add the noodles to the simmering soup. Cook one minute.

Add the chicken to the soup. Add the lemon juice, green onion, salt, and pepper. Cook for one minute. Pour into bowls. Add a squeeze of lime or lemon juice and some chopped cilantro. Serve.

───────────────── ❧ ─────────────────

Serves 8

*Information on this ingredient is included in the Glossary.

SPICY SEAFOOD SOUP
Quick and Adventurous

282 calories per serving

Prep Time: 15 minutes
Cook Time: 30 minutes

1 onion, chopped
1 clove garlic, chopped
3 chilies (jalapeno or serrano*),
    seeded and sliced
1 Tbsp. peanut oil
4 cups homemade chicken stock
    (see recipe on page 132)
    or canned nonfat broth
2 cups fish stock* (or clam juice)
3 cups water
2 potatoes, cut into $1/2$-inch cubes

1 package enoki mushrooms*
$1/2$ cup rice (uncooked)
1 bunch cilantro,* chopped
$1/4$ cup lemon juice
4 stalks lemon grass,*
    peeled and sliced
4 slices galanga,* soaked in
    water for 10 minutes
1 Tbsp. fish sauce*
1 Tbsp. rice vinegar
1 tsp. soy sauce

$1/3$ lb. scallops
$3/4$ lb. shrimp, peeled
6–8 "littleneck" clams

─────────────── ❧ ───────────────

Heat the oil. Saute the onion, garlic, and chilies until the onion is slightly transparent. Add the rest of the ingredients, except the seafood. Simmer for 20 minutes, covered. Add the seafood, and cook 5 minutes longer. Serve.

─────────────── ❧ ───────────────

Serves 6

Please don't be discouraged by the number of ingredients in this recipe. This is a wonderful soup that is a meal in itself. Galanga has no substitute; if you can't find it in an Asian store, leave it out. The recipe will still be delicious.

*Information on this ingredient is included in the Glossary.

First-Course
and
Main-Dish
Salads

TOSTADA SALAD
Adventurous

338 calories per serving

Prep Time: 30 minutes
Cook Time: 5 minutes

> 3–4 cups mixed salad greens
> 1 cup cooked black beans, canned or homemade (see
>   Basic Black Bean Recipe on page 223)
> $1/2$ cup cooked corn kernels
> $1/3$ cup celery, diced
> 1 cup salsa (see Traditional Salsa recipe on page 159)
> salt and pepper to taste

> **Dressing:**
> $1/2$ cup cooked beans (canned or fresh)
> $1/4$ clove garlic
> 4 tsp. balsamic vinegar

Puree the dressing ingredients in a blender or food processor. Toss the dressing with the salad greens and celery. Arrange the dressed greens on a plate. Put a scoop (about $1/2$ cup) of salsa in the middle. Toss the other beans and corn together with salt and pepper, and scatter over the greens.

Optional: Cut a corn tortilla into pie-wedge pieces and toast in a 400-degree oven until crisp and brown. Stick a few pieces upright in the salad for visual impact and added crunch. And add a spoonful of fat-free sour cream if you'd like.

Serves 2 as a luncheon salad.

First-Course and Main-Dish Salads

POTATO SALAD
Easy

135 calories per serving

Prep Time: 15 minutes
Cook Time: 15–25 minutes

1¹/2 lbs. red potatoes, peeled, diced
2 stalks celery, thinly sliced
3 eggs, hardboiled
4 Tbsp. green onions, chopped
4 Tbsp. parsley, chopped
1 Tbsp. Dijon mustard
2 Tbsp. sweet pickle relish
3 Tbsp. wine vinegar
1 Tbsp. vegetable oil
1/2 cup fat-free sour cream
1/2 tsp. sugar
salt and pepper to taste

Boil the potatoes until fork tender, drain well in a colander, and sprinkle with 2 tablespoons of vinegar, salt, and pepper. Combine the other ingredients. To keep this really low fat, throw the yolks of the eggs away, and chop the whites. Combine with all other ingredients. Mix well and toss with potatoes. Allow to chill so that flavors have a chance to blend.

Serves 6

CREAMY SLAW
Quick and Easy

25 calories per serving

Prep Time: 10 minutes
Cook Time: 0

$1/2$ head cabbage or Napa cabbage, sliced and shredded

Dressing:
1 clove garlic, chopped
1 Tbsp. green onion, chopped (green part only)
$1/4$ tsp. salt
$1/4$ tsp. pepper
$1/2$ tsp. sugar (or sugar substitute)
2 Tbsp. red wine vinegar
1 Tbsp. lemon juice
$1/2$ tsp. mustard seed
$1/2$ cup fat-free sour cream or fat-free plain yogurt
1 tsp. vegetable oil

———————————— ❦ ————————————

Whisk together dressing ingredients. Toss with cabbage. Allow to rest at least 15 minutes before serving so that flavors can blend.

———————————— ❦ ————————————

Serves 6

*This slaw makes a perfect accompaniment
to a barbeque dish. It is especially good on
barbeque turkey sandwiches.*

First-Course and Main-Dish Salads

FRUIT SALAD
Quick and Easy

118 calories per serving

Prep Time: 10 minutes
Cook Time: 0

> 2 persimmons, sliced
> 10 kumquats, sliced
> 1 banana, sliced
> 3–4 sprigs of mint, chopped
> juice of one orange
> "juice" from 2 inches fresh ginger

Grate the ginger into a bowl and, with your fingers, squeeze out the liquid into the orange juice. Combine the persimmons, kumquats, and banana with the mint. Add the juice and mix. Serve cool or at room temperature.

Serves 2–4 as a salad or a dessert

First-Course and Main-Dish Salads

SALAD OF GRAPEFRUIT, ORANGE, FENNEL, AND FIELD GREENS
Quick and Easy

96 calories per serving

Prep Time: 10 minutes
Cook Time: 0

> 2 small grapefruits, sectioned, with membranes removed
> 1 large orange, sectioned, with membranes removed
> juice of $1/2$ orange
> juice of $1/2$ grapefruit
> $1/2$ fennel bulb, sliced
> 3 cups assorted salad greens or frisee lettuce
> 1 shallot, chopped
> $1/2$ tsp. salt
> $1/4$ tsp. pepper
> 1 Tbsp. olive oil

Combine the juices with the shallot, salt, pepper, and oil. Blend well. You will have a very loose emulsion. Combine the grapefruit, orange, fennel, and salad greens, and mix well. Mix with the "vinaigrette" and divide onto plates. Serve with a grind of fresh black pepper.

Serves 4

COLE SLAW WITH CELERY SEED VINAIGRETTE

Quick and Easy

38 calories per serving

Prep Time: 15 minutes
Cook Time: 0
Marinate Time: 30 or more minutes

1 lb. cabbage, cored and sliced

4 Tbsp. red wine vinegar
1 tsp. canola or vegetable oil
$1/4$ tsp. sesame oil
$1/2$ tsp. celery seed
$1/2$ tsp. salt
$3/4$ tsp. ground black pepper
2 tsp. sugar
3 Tbsp. green onions, green part only, chopped
3 Tbsp. parsley, chopped
1 Tbsp. lemon juice

———————————— ❧ ————————————

Whisk together all ingredients, except cabbage, until well combined. Toss with cabbage. Refrigerate and serve.

———————————— ❧ ————————————

Serves 6

GREEN PINEAPPLE SALAD
Quick and Easy

58 calories per serving

Prep Time: 10 minutes
Cook Time: 0

      1 stalk celery, chopped
      1 $1/2$ cups salad greens, loosely packed, dry
      1 cup diced pineapple
      6 asparagus spears, steamed 5–7 minutes
      1 green onion, chopped
      $1/8$ red onion, sliced
      $1/2$ tsp. Dijon mustard
      $1/8$ tsp. pepper
      salt to taste
      $1 1/2$ Tbsp. balsamic vinegar
      $1/4$ cup pureed raspberries

Combine all of the ingredients and mix well.

Serves 2

TEX-MEX SALAD
Quick and Adventurous

163 calories per serving

Prep Time: 15 minutes
Cook Time: 7 minutes (for squash)

> 1 chayote squash, peeled, cored, and cubed
> 1 cup jicama,* peeled and cubed
> 1 tomato, diced
> 1 jalapeno chili,* seeded and minced
> 2 Tbsp. red onion, chopped
> 4 Tbsp. fresh cilantro,* chopped
> 2 sundried tomatoes, chopped
> 2 Tbsp. lime juice
> 1 Tbsp. olive oil
> salt and pepper to taste
>
> 2–4 romaine lettuce leaves

Steam the chayote squash until tender, about 5–7 minutes. Cool. Combine lime juice, oil, salt, and pepper. Mix well. Toss with all other ingredients. Serve on romaine leaves at room temperature or chilled.

Serves 2

*Information on this ingredient is included in the Glossary.

BERKELEY SALAD
Quick and Adventurous

80 calories per serving

Prep Time: 15 minutes
Cook Time: 0

$^1/_4$ small jicama,* julienned
1 fresh Anaheim chili,* chopped
1 fresh pasilla chili,* chopped
1 Japanese (or regular) cucumber, sliced
1 tomato, seeded and diced
1 yellow squash (crook-neck/swan-neck), chopped
1 small bunch cilantro,* chopped

Dressing: (makes $^1/_3$ cup)
1 sundried tomato
2 Tbsp. olive oil
$^1/_2$ lemon, peeled, seeded, and chopped
$^1/_8$ tsp. salt
$^1/_8$ tsp. pepper
1 pinch sugar

Combine all dressing ingredients in a blender, and blend until fully emulsified. Combine the salad ingredients and toss with 3–4 tablespoons dressing. (The remaining dressing can be kept in the refrigerator for several days. Use it on a green salad.)

Serves 4

*Information on this ingredient is included in the Glossary.

First-Course and Main-Dish Salads

TABBOULEH
Adventurous

35 calories per serving

Prep Time: 30 minutes
Cook Time: 0

1 cup uncooked bulgur wheat*
2 cups water
1 red onion, chopped fine
1 bunch parsley, chopped fine (flat leaf parsley is best for this)
1 red or green pepper, chopped fine
1 cucumber, seeded and chopped fine
2 tomatoes, seeded and chopped fine
3 Tbsp. mint, chopped fine
1 jalapeno chili,* chopped fine
2 Tbsp. garlic, chopped fine
1 tsp. salt
1/2 tsp. black pepper
1/3 cup lemon juice

Bring water to a boil, and pour over bulgur wheat. Allow to soak while you chop the vegetables (at least 15 minutes). Drain the wheat well and toss with all the other ingredients. Taste for seasoning.

Serves 12 as an appetizer,
or 8 as a salad

This great dish makes a wonderful low-fat appetizer. Serve it in a large bowl surrounded with romaine leaves with a little bowl of hummus on the side. Spoon a little hummus on a romaine leaf. Top with tabbouleh. Roll up the leaf and eat with your hands. Tabbouleh also makes a good vegetarian sandwich served in pita bread with a little hummus and some lettuce.

*Information on this ingredient is included in the Glossary.

STEAMED ARTICHOKE STUFFED WITH SHRIMP OR CRAB SALAD

Quick and Easy

122 calories per serving

Prep Time: 10 minutes
Cook Time: 0–10 minutes

4–8 oz. cooked shrimp or crab
2 artichokes

Dressing: (makes one cup)
4 Tbsp. HoMade Chili Sauce (HoMade is our favorite
    brand; it is sweet, not spicy). You may, of course,
    substitute your favorite.
2 tsp. Dijon mustard
1 clove garlic, chopped
1 stalk celery, chopped
2 green onions, green part only, chopped
2 Tbsp. parsley, chopped
1 tsp. horseradish
4 Tbsp. nonfat sour cream
$1/4$ tsp. sugar
2 Tbsp. lemon juice

Optional: If you like a thinner consistency, add 1–2 tablespoons wine vinegar

———————————— ❧ ————————————

Combine the dressing ingredients and set aside.
Steam the artichokes. Remove the choke when artichoke has cooled slightly
by pulling apart the inner leaves and removing them. Then take a spoon and carefully remove the bristly choke. You will be left with an intact artichoke open in the
center, where you're able to see the heart.
Combine $1/2$ cup dressing (more or less to your liking) with shellfish. Spoon
into artichoke and serve. Make sure not to skimp on the dressing. You and your
guest(s) will end up using it to dip the artichoke leaves in.

———————————— ❧ ————————————

Serves 2

This salad is also great served in a half cantaloupe or just
tossed will salad greens.

THAI SHRIMP AND RICE NOODLE SALAD
Quick and Easy

292 calories per serving

Prep Time: 15 minutes
Cook Time: 5 minutes

    4 oz. rice noodles
    2 tsp. sesame oil
    8 ounces Napa cabbage (one cabbage), chopped
    12 oz. shrimp
    $1/2$ cup lemon juice (lime is even better)
    $1/4$ cup fish sauce*
    1 clove garlic, crushed
    3 green onions, sliced
    "heat"

Steam or boil the dry rice noodles until soft. Toss with the sesame oil and save. Peel and slice the shrimp in half. Combine the lemon juice, fish sauce, garlic, and "heat."

In a wok, saute the shrimp in one teaspoon oil until almost done. Add the Napa cabbage and stir well. Add half the lemon and fish sauce mixture, and stir well. When cabbage starts to wilt, add the noodles and mix. Add the rest of the sauce. If too strong for your taste, add up to one cup water. Ladle into bowls, garnish with chives, cilantro, or flat parsley, and serve.

Serves 4

*Information on this ingredient is included in the Glossary.

First-Course and Main-Dish Salads

SQUID SALAD

Adventurous

276 calories per serving

Prep Time: 15 minutes
Cook Time: 60 minutes
    (if you use canned beans, cook time is about 10 minutes)

1 cup dry black beans
    (or 2 cups canned, drained)
4 cups water
1 small onion, quartered
4 cloves
2 bay leaves
2 cloves garlic
1 dry red chili
$^1/_2$ firm mango, diced
2 Tbsp. cilantro,* chopped
2 Tbsp. red wine vinegar
salt and pepper to taste
$^2/_3$ lb. cleaned squid, sliced

Dressing:
1 Tbsp. olive oil
2 shallots, sliced
1 clove garlic, chopped
1 jalapeno* or serrano* chili, minced
4 Tbsp. lemon juice
1 Tbsp. cilantro,* chopped

You may prepare the dressing and soak the beans ahead of time. To prepare the dressing, whisk together the lemon juice and oil until well blended. Add the other ingredients and mix well. Refrigerate until needed.

For the beans: Bring water to boil, add the beans, and turn off the heat. Let the beans sit for an hour (or overnight). After soaking, drain the beans. Bring 4 cups of water to a boil. Lower the heat to a simmer. Stick the cloves in the onion and add to the water, along with the bay leaves, red chili, 2 cloves garlic, and the beans. Simmer, covered, until the beans are tender, about one hour. If you use canned beans, cook 15 minutes.

Remove the onion, chili, bay leaves, and garlic. Discard cloves. Chop the onion. Drain the beans, and toss them with the mango, cilantro, vinegar, salt, and pepper. Cook the squid in boiling water for 3 minutes. Drain and toss with the dressing.

To serve: Place the bean mixture in a thin layer all over each plate. Top with a mound of squid salad in the middle. Sprinkle with cilantro.

Serves 4

*Information on this ingredient is included in the Glossary.

AHI (TUNA) SALAD
Quick and Easy

256 calories per serving

Prep Time: 10 minutes
Cook Time: 10 minutes

1 lb. fresh tuna
1 cup fava beans
$1/2$ small head radicchio, chopped
2 bunches arugula, chopped
2 bunches watercress, chopped
$1/2$ red onion, sliced

Dressing:
5 tsp. lime juice
3 Tbsp. olive oil
$1/4$ tsp. dry mustard
$1/8$ tsp. ground pepper
$1/4$ tsp. sugar or honey (optional)
salt to taste (optional)

Grill tuna (ahi) in nonstick pan sprayed first with vegetable spray. The tuna will take about 2–3 minutes per side depending on its thickness and how hot you can get your pan. It should be cooked medium rare.

Shell the fava beans and cook in boiling water until they are tender, about 4 minutes. Cool and remove their outer skin.

Mix the dressing ingredients well, until emulsified. Toss with salad ingredients. Slice the ahi tuna in $3/4$ inch slices, and arrange artfully on top of the salad.

Serve at room temperature.

Serves 4

*Information on this ingredient is included in the Glossary.

CHINESE CHICKEN SALAD

Quick and Easy

460 calories per serving

Prep Time: 20 minutes
Cook Time: 10 minutes

2 chicken breasts, boneless and skinless

Marinade:
1–2 cloves garlic, pressed through garlic press (or chopped)
1 Tbsp. soy sauce
$1/4$ tsp. ground black pepper
$1/4$ tsp. sesame oil

———————————————— ❧ ————————————————

Slice chicken into strips about 1 inch wide. Combine marinade ingredients and pour over chicken. Marinate for 15 minutes while making the rest of the salad.

———————————————— ❧ ————————————————

Salad Dressing:
1 Tbsp. sugar
$1/4$ tsp. salt
$1/4$ tsp. ground black pepper
3 Tbsp. red wine vinegar or rice wine vinegar*
1 Tbsp. vegetable oil
$1/4$ tsp. sesame oil
Optional: 2 pieces 5-star anise

———————————————— ❧ ————————————————

Whisk together salad ingredients until well combined. Allow to sit at least 10 minutes so that flavors can combine. May be made a day ahead.

CHINESE CHICKEN SALAD (CONT.)

1 bunch romaine (or head lettuce)
1 carrot cut into strips (I just peel it with a potato peeler)
4 green onions, cut on the diagonal into 1" pieces
$^1/_2$ cup Chinese parsley (cilantro), slightly chopped
$^1/_2$ Tbsp. sesame seeds
1 Tbsp. fresh ginger cut into strips (I use the potato peeler)
1 handful (that's $^1/_4$ cup when softened in
     water) of rice sticks or bean threads

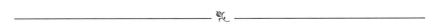

Soak the rice sticks in hot water for about 5 minutes or until softened. Drain and allow to dry slightly on paper towels. In a nonstick pan, dry-fry the rice sticks until slightly brown, about 3 or 4 minutes. Set aside. In the same pan, quickly saute the chicken until brown on both sides, about 2 minutes on each side.

Toss the romaine, carrot, cilantro, green onions, and ginger with the salad dressing. Arrange on large plates. Sprinkle with sesame seeds. Arrange the chicken strips like spokes of a wheel. Top with rice sticks and serve.

Serves 4 as a main course

LOBSTER AND ARTICHOKE SALAD

Quick and Easy

80 calories per serving

Prep Time: 10 minutes
Cook Time: 0

$2^1/2$ oz. lobster meat
$2^1/2$ oz. artichoke hearts, in cubes
2 tsp. green chili (or pepper), chopped
1 Tbsp. green onion, chopped
6 cups salad greens
1 tsp. truffle oil*
1 tsp. lemon juice

Shallot Vinaigrette:
1 Tbsp. shallots, chopped
$1/4$ tsp. salt
$1/4$ tsp. pepper
2 Tbsp. lemon juice
4 tsp. walnut oil

———————— ❧ ————————

You can prepare this salad if you have some lobster and artichokes left-over from another recipe (such as the Lobster and Artichoke Soup recipe on page 192).

Combine the lobster, artichoke hearts, chili (or ground pepper), and the green onion with one teaspoon truffle oil and one teaspoon lemon juice. Mix well.

Prepare the shallot vinaigrette: Put the shallots, salt, and pepper in a bowl. Add the tablespoon of lemon juice and beat with a whisk. Add the oil in portions, whisking furiously. Add the salad greens (baby romaine would be best here). Place on four plates, and divide the lobster artichoke mixture on top of the greens.

———————— ❧ ————————

Serves 4

*Information on this ingredient is included in the Glossary

Vegetables, Pasta, and Risottos

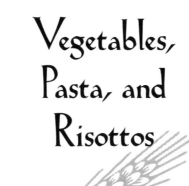

CORN-STUFFED CHILIES
Adventurous

95 calories per serving

Prep Time: 20 minutes
Cook Time: 15–20 minutes

> 4 fresh Anaheim* or pasilla* chilies (about 4 oz. each)
> 4 Tbsp. red onion, chopped
> 4 Tbsp. cilantro, chopped
> 1^{1}/2 cups corn kernels (frozen or fresh); if fresh, parboil
>   for 2 minutes
> ^{1}/2 cup mock cheese (optional—see recipe on page 318)
> ^{1}/4 tsp. salt

Parboil chilies until slightly soft, about 6 minutes. Cool. Carefully remove stem and cap with a knife. Shake out seeds. Combine other ingredients and carefully stuff them into the peppers. Replace caps. Cook stuffed chilies under broiler or in a 400-degree oven, turning them as they brown so that all sides are cooked. They will take about 15–20 minutes to cook depending on the heat and the size of the chilies.

Serves 4

Serve this dish with fruit salsa. The contrast of the sweet salsa and the spicy chilies makes a great combination.

*Information on this ingredient is included in the Glossary.

Vegetables, Pasta, and Risottos

3-SQUASH SQUASH
Quick and Easy

77 calories per serving

Prep Time: 15 minutes
Cook Time: 15–20 minutes

1 onion, chopped
2 cloves garlic, chopped
1 stalk celery, chopped
2 small zucchini, sliced
2 yellow crookneck squash, sliced
3 summer squash, cubed
2 tsp. curry powder*
$1/4$ tsp. ground cumin*
$1/4$ tsp. turmeric*
$1/2$ to 1 cup water
$1/4$ tsp. sugar
$1/4$ tsp. ground black pepper
$1/2$ tsp. salt
1 Asian pear (or an apple or a pear), peeled,
    seeded, and chopped
1 Tbsp. lemon juice

Spray a nonstick skillet with vegetable spray. Heat. Add curry, cumin, and turmeric, and stir, cooking over low heat for 1–2 minutes until well blended and the aroma fills your kitchen. Add onion, garlic, and celery and cook 7–8 minutes, stirring frequently. Add a half cup water, and mix well with ingredients in the skillet. Add all the squash, salt, pepper, and sugar. Mix well, lower heat and simmer, covered, for 8 minutes. Stir occasionally, and when all the liquid is absorbed, add additional water. Uncovered, raise heat to medium, add apple or pear, and cook until most liquid is absorbed and what is left is thickened (about 2–3 minutes). Sprinkle with lemon juice and serve.

Serves 4

*Information on this ingredient is included in the Glossary.

Vegetables, Pasta, and Risottos

MISSISSIPPI YAMS
Quick and Easy

167 calories per serving

Prep Time: 20 minutes
Cook Time: 30 minutes

2 lbs. yams
$1/2$ tsp. salt
$1/4$ cup brown sugar (or maple syrup)
$1/4$–$1/2$ cup bourbon (to taste)
$1/4$ cup raisins
1 tsp. lemon juice
3–4 oz. pineapple, chopped
2 tsp. vegetable oil

Boil the yams until soft when pricked with a fork, about 15–20 minutes. While the yams are boiling, combine the brown sugar, bourbon, and raisins in a saucepan and cook over low heat for 3–5 minutes, until the raisins are plumped and the alcohol has evaporated. Remove the skin from the yams (it should practically fall off), and mash the yams. Combine the yams, salt, pineapple, and lemon juice, with the sugar, bourbon, and raisin mixture. If you prefer, you may add a sugar substitute for more sweetness. When ready to serve, heat in a 350-degree oven for 20 minutes.

Serves 8

This is a wonderful accompaniment to turkey, chicken, or other fowl. It can be made up to two days ahead and freezes well. It's great for the Thanksgiving and Christmas holidays.

Vegetables, Pasta, and Risottos

SWEET AND SOUR EGGPLANT
Quick and Adventurous

193 calories per serving

Prep Time: 15 minutes
Cook Time: 25 minutes

$1^1/_2$ tsp. ground coriander*
$1^1/_2$ tsp. ground cumin*
$1/_2$ tsp. ground fenugreek*
1 tsp. ground turmeric*
1 Tbsp. mustard oil*
1 onion, chopped
1 jalapeno chili,* chopped
$1/_4$ cup lime juice
$1/_4$ cup maple syrup
3 Japanese eggplants,* chopped
3 tomatoes, seeded and chopped
2 Tbsp. fresh cilantro,* chopped
1 Tbsp. vinegar
$1/_2$ cup water

———————————————— ✻ ————————————————

Heat the oil. When it smokes, add the ground coriander, cumin, fenu-greek, and turmeric. Cook until they begin to smell pungent. Brown the spices; do not burn! Add the onion and chili. Cook on low heat, stirring fre-quently, about 4 minutes. Add $1/_4$ cup water and continue cooking until the onion is soft, about 6 minutes. Add the lime juice, vinegar, and maple syrup. Cook for 4–5 minutes over low heat, stirring frequently. Add the eggplant, tomatoes, two tablespoons cilantro, and $1/_4$ cup water. Stir, cover, and sim-mer for 5 minutes. Remove the cover and continue cooking for 5 minutes or until eggplant is fork tender. Add more water if the mixture becomes too dry. Serve very hot.

———————————————— ✻ ————————————————

Serves 4

This recipe is great served with meat,
fish, or fowl, or alone as a vegetarian dish.

*Information on this ingredient is included in the Glossary.

SONORA AUBERGINES
Adventurous

244 calories per serving

Prep Time: 25 minutes
Cook Time: 20 minutes (eggplant); 25 minutes (whole dish)

> 1 eggplant
> 8 fava bean pods
> 1 dry pasilla chili*
> 1 dry New Mexico chili*
> 2 cups water
> 1 tomato, peeled, seeded, and chopped
> 1 onion, chopped
> 1 clove garlic, chopped
> 1 tomatillo,* diced
> 1 tsp. ground cumin
> 2 Tbsp. honey
> 2 tsp. olive oil
> juice of one lemon
> $^1/4$ tsp. salt

───────────────── ❧ ─────────────────

Cut the eggplant in half, and place, cut side down, on a nonstick surface. Bake in a 250-degree oven for 20 minutes, or until soft. Cool, peel, and chop.

Soak the chilies in the water while the eggplant cooks, then puree the chilies in blender using 1–2 tablespoons of soaking water. Save the rest of the soaking water.

Shell fava beans. Parboil for two minutes. Remove the tough outer skin from each bean.

Heat the oil. Cook onion, garlic, chilies, tomatillo, and cumin over low heat until onion is transparent (about 5 minutes). Add the tomato and honey. Stir to incorporate. Add the fava beans, eggplant, and the remaining water in which you soaked the chilies. Stir, cover, and cook on low heat for 20 minutes, stirring occasionally. Add lemon juice and salt. Stir until well combined. Serve.

───────────────── ❧ ─────────────────

Serves 4

*Information on this ingredient is included in the Glossary.

RATATOUILLE
Quick and Easy

Vegetables, Pasta, and Risottos

81 calories per serving

Prep Time: 20 minutes
Cook Time: 20 minutes

1 onion
2 cloves garlic (4 cloves, if you really like garlic)
1 jalapeno chili,* seeded
1 Japanese eggplant*
1 zucchini
1 summer squash
1 yellow zucchini (or crook neck) squash
1 red bell pepper, seeded and de-veined
2 tomatoes, seeded and cored
1 tsp. oregano, chopped
$^1/_4$ tsp. salt
$^1/_4$ tsp. sugar (optional)
1 Tbsp. olive oil
$^1/_2$ cup water
$^1/_4$ tsp. ground pepper (or to taste)

Dice all of the vegetables. (You may combine the squashes in one bowl, but keep the other vegetables separate.) Spray a nonstick pan with vegetable oil and heat. Add onion, garlic, and chili, and cook on low heat until slightly brown. Add the red pepper and continue cooking until the pepper is slightly soft (about 5 minutes). As the ingredients in the pan begin to dry, start adding the water, a tablespoon at a time, throughout the rest of the cooking. Add the squashes and cook until "al dente" (about 5 minutes). Add the eggplant and cook for two minutes. Finally, add the tomato, oregano, salt, sugar, and pepper, and cook for 2–3 minutes.

Serves 4

May be made two days ahead. It actually gets better with time. May be served hot, cold, or at room temperature. This is great as a vegetarian dish, but it is also fun to use as a stuffing for poultry.

Ron firmly believes the vegetables should be hand diced, not chopped in the food processor. If you dice everything very small, this also makes a great filling for zucchini blossoms.

Kathye is responsible for the optional sugar. She believes a pinch of sugar brings out the natural sweetness in vegetables, especially tomatoes, and substantially enhances the taste.

*Information on this ingredient is included in the Glossary.

VEGETABLE CURRY
Quick and Easy

223 calories per serving

Prep Time: 15 minutes
Cook Time: 15 minutes

1 Tbsp. mustard oil* (or vegetable oil)
1 onion, chopped
3 cloves garlic, chopped
2–4 tsp. curry powder (depending on your taste)
1 ear of corn, kernels removed
1 summer squash, chopped
1 swan neck squash, chopped
1 yellow bell pepper, diced
4 small red potatoes, parboiled and cubed
2 Japanese eggplants* (or $^1/_2$ regular eggplant), cubed
1 cup mushrooms, sliced
$^1/_2$ cup tomato sauce
1 cup homemade chicken or vegetable stock (see recipes
    on page 131–132) or canned nonfat broth
2 Tbsp. parsley, chopped
juice of $^1/_2$ lime (or lemon)
salt and pepper to taste

Heat the oil. Add the onion, garlic, and curry powder, and saute until translucent. Add the rest of the ingredients in the following order, stirring after each addition: corn, squash, bell pepper, potatoes, eggplant, mushrooms, tomato sauce, stock, parsley, and lime juice. Cook until tender (6–8 minutes), adding more stock if mixture becomes too dry. Add salt and pepper to taste.

Serves 4

*Information on this ingredient is included in the Glossary.

Vegetables, Pasta, and Risottos

BASIC BLACK BEAN RECIPE

Easy

167 calories per serving

Prep Time: 15 minutes
Cook Time: 60 minutes plus presoak

> 1 lb. package dry black (turtle) beans
> 7 cups water
> 1 onion, quartered
> 2 cloves garlic, cut in halves
> 1 bay leaf
> 2 cloves
> 1 tsp. dried oregano
> $1/2$ tsp. cumin seeds*
> 3 Tbsp. apple cider or wine vinegar
> $1^1/2$ tsp. salt
> $1/2$ tsp. ground black pepper
> $1/2$ tsp. sugar

Soak the beans ahead of time, either overnight in a bowl of water or by pouring 4 cups of boiling water over them and soaking for one hour.

After soaking, add the beans to a large pot with the water, onion, garlic, bay leaf, cloves, oregano, and cumin seeds. Bring to a simmer; cover and cook for 45 minutes.

After cooking, add the apple cider or wine vinegar, salt, pepper, and sugar. Continue cooking uncovered until the beans are tender. Taste to see if additional salt or pepper is needed.

This basic black bean recipe is for use when beans are called for as an ingredient in a recipe such as Bean Dip or Tostada Salad.

Serves 8–12 if using as a side dish

*Information on this ingredient is included in the Glossary.

SMOKED BEAN STEW WITH SAUERKRAUT
Easy

107 calories per serving

Prep Time: 5 minutes
Cook time: 60 minutes, plus presoak

$^1/_2$ cup dry great northern beans
4 ounces sauerkraut
1 Tbsp. balsamic vinegar
$1^1/_2$ cups homemade chicken or vegetable stock (see
recipe on pages 131–132) or canned nonfat broth

Soak the beans ahead of time, either overnight in a bowl of water or by pouring 4 cups of boiling water over them and soaking for one hour. Cook in unsalted water until tender. Drain. Smoke the beans on a covered screen grid for 15 minutes. Combine the beans with the rest of the ingredients in a pot, heat through and serve.

Serves 4

Good with lean sliced pork tenderloin.

Vegetables, Pasta, and Risottos

GRILLED PORTOBELLO MUSHROOMS

Quick and Easy

156 calories per serving

Prep Time: 10 minutes
Cook Time: 10 minutes

4 portobello mushrooms*
1 Tbsp. olive oil
1 clove garlic, chopped

Sauce:
1 cup homemade chicken or vegetable stock
    (see recipes on pages 131–132) or canned nonfat broth
$^1/_2$ cup red wine
1 shallot, chopped
2 tsp. smoked pork or ham, chopped fine (optional)
$1^1/_2$ cups corn
$^1/_4$ cup brandy
2 Tbsp. parsley
salt and pepper to taste

Heat a nonstick pan. Add oil, then garlic and mushrooms. Saute mushrooms on both sides until done (about 5 minutes per side). Remove mushrooms to warm dish. Add brandy to pan and deglaze (scrap up any particles sticking to the bottom). When liquid is absorbed, add pork, wine, shallot, chicken broth, and one tablespoon of the parsley. Boil, stirring frequently until sauce begins to thicken (about 3–5 minutes). Add corn, and simmer 3 minutes. Add salt and pepper to taste. Spoon sauce, with corn on the bottom of each plate. Place a mushroom in the middle (whole or sliced). Sprinkle with rest of parsley and serve.

Serves 4

*Information on this ingredient is included in the Glossary.

Vegetables, Pasta, and Risottos

WILD MUSHROOM SANDWICH ON CARAWAY POLENTA TOAST

Adventurous

138 calories per serving

Prep Time: 20 minutes
Cook Time: 20 minutes

> 1 cup polenta (corn meal)
> 4 cups water
> 2 Tbsp. caraway seeds*
> $^1/_4$ tsp. salt
> $^3/_4$ cup dried morel mushrooms*
> 3 crimini mushrooms,* sliced
> 2 large shiitake mushrooms,* sliced
> 1 small portobello mushroom,* sliced
> $^1/_2$ onion chopped
> 1 serrano chili*
> 3 cloves garlic, chopped
> 2 Tbsp. chopped shallots
> 1 Tbsp. walnut oil
> lemon juice
> $^1/_4$ cup brandy or cognac
> chopped parsley for garnish
> salt and pepper to taste

Make the polenta: Combine one cup polenta with 4 cups of water, 2 tablespoons caraway seeds and salt. Stir well and bring to a boil. Reduce heat and stir occasionally, making sure it does not burn or stick on the bottom of the pan. Taste for consistency. When the polenta is soft with no hard granules, turn the polenta onto an oiled, smooth flat surface (such as a pastry board) and, using a spatula, spread it to an even thickness of a little less than $^3/_4$" thick.

*Information on this ingredient is included in the Glossary.

WILD MUSHROOM SANDWICH (CONT.)

While the polenta is cooling, make the mushrooms: Soak the morels and the rest of the mushrooms in about 3 cups of water. When the morels are soft, take them out of the water, cut them in halves, and rinse under running water. Add the sliced morels and the rest of the mushrooms back to the liquid and steep until soft. Remove the mushrooms and strain the liquid off the sand on the bottom. In a saucepan, heat one tablespoon walnut oil and saute the onion, garlic, shallots, and chili until nicely tan. Add all of the mushrooms and stir well. Pour in $1/4$ cup brandy and flame. When the fire in the pan dies down, add the soaking liquid (you will have about 2 cups). Bring to a simmer and carefully skim off all the oil rising to the surface. Cook for about 10 minutes until the liquid starts to have some consistency. Taste and correct the seasoning by adding a squirt of lemon juice, salt, and pepper as necessary. Keep it warm but not boiling.

Slice the polenta into 4-by-4-inch squares and then cut them on one diagonal to make triangles. You will have at least 18 triangles. Saute these in a nonstick pan with a tiny amount of oil until they are "toasted." Make a single- or double-decker sandwich by spooning the mushrooms over polenta and covering with another slice. Sprinkle on parsley for color, and serve.

Makes 4–6 main courses or about 8 appetizers

Vegetables, Pasta, and Risottos

VEGETABLE COUSCOUS
Quick and Easy

97 calories per serving

Prep Time: 15 minutes
Cook Time: 10 minutes

1¹/₂ cups cooked couscous* (to cook: follow instructions on box)
1 crook neck squash,* chopped
1¹/₂ summer squash, chopped
1 small zucchini, chopped
1 clove garlic, chopped
¹/₂ cup homemade nonfat vegetable or chicken stock
    (see recipes on pages 131–132) or canned nonfat broth
¹/₂ cup water
Optional: ¹/₂ tsp. harissa*

Combine all ingredients, except couscous, in an uncovered saucepan, and boil until vegetables are cooked, but still crisp. Most of the liquid will have boiled away. Add couscous and harissa, mix well, and continue cooking until heated through. Serve.

Serves 4

*Information on this ingredient is included in the Glossary.

Vegetables, Pasta, and Risottos

FRUIT COUSCOUS
Quick and Easy

138 calories per serving

Prep Time: 10 minutes
Cook Time: 10 minutes

> $1^1/2$ cooked couscous* (to cook, follow instructions on box)
> $^1/2$ cup mixed dried fruit, chopped
> $^1/4$ cup raisins
> $^1/2$ cup water
> $^1/2$ cup homemade nonfat vegetable or chicken stock
>   (see recipes on pages 131-132) or canned nonfat broth
> 1 tsp. lemon or lime juice
> 1 stick cinnamon

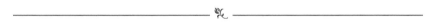

Combine all ingredients, except couscous, in a saucepan. Boil for 10 minutes or until fruit has softened and raisins have plumped. Most of the liquid will have boiled away. Add couscous, stir carefully, lower heat, and continue cooking until heated through. Remove cinnamon stick. Serve.

Serves 4

CREAMY POLENTA
Quick and Easy

140 calories per serving

Prep Time: 2 minutes
Cook Time: 20 minutes

  4 cups boiling water
  2 tsp. salt
  1^1/2 cups yellow corn meal mixed with 2 cups water
  1 cup nonfat milk

In a separate bowl, mix the corn meal with the water until it is well combined and not lumpy. If lumpiness persists, add more water until it is smooth. Add this mixture gradually to the boiling water, stirring constantly. Continue cooking over moderate heat, stirring almost constantly. As the water begins to get absorbed, lower the heat, and very slowly add the milk and salt. It should take at least 20 minutes to thoroughly cook the corn meal and get to the right creamy texture. If it is cooking too fast, lower your heat and add more water.

Serves 6–8

This is such an easy recipe that we almost didn't include it. So many of our friends have asked how we made our polenta creamy instead of the traditional solid, we thought we'd let you know.

Vegetables, Pasta, and Risottos

CURRIED LENTILS
Quick and Adventurous

370 calories per serving

Prep Time: 10 minutes
Cook Time: 20 minutes (depends on type of lentils)

1 cup lentils (see note below) washed in cold water and
    then placed in bowl with water to cover
2 tsp. cumin,* ground
2 tsp. coriander,* ground
$1/2$ tsp. turmeric,* ground
$1/8$ tsp. asafoetida,* ground
10 curry leaves*
1 medium onion, chopped
ground cayenne to taste (pinch or two)
$1/8$ tsp. salt
water
2 tsp. mustard oil* (or vegetable, olive, or canola oil)
1 Tbsp. lemon juice (about $1/2$ a small lemon)
pepper to taste

—————————————— ❧ ——————————————

In a heavy saucepan of at least 8 cups capacity, heat the mustard oil. Add the ground spices, except the cayenne, and stir until they turn from light shades of brown to dark brown. Don't let them burn, but they must be cooked in the oil to release their flavors. Quickly add the chopped onion and stir well. Add the curry leaves and cayenne. Stir until the onion is just starting to turn golden, and then add the DRAINED lentils and two cups of water. Stir well, bring back to a simmer, and cook until the lentils are done. (They should be firm but not hard, soft but not mushy.) The water will be almost totally absorbed. Depending on the type of lentils used, you may need more water. Taste for salt and add some ($1/8$ teaspoon) if required. Add the lemon juice and stir well. Taste again for salt, citrus, and pepper, and add as needed.

—————————————— ❧ ——————————————

Serves 2 as a generous side dish

Chefs' note: It's possible to make this recipe with only the lentils, some prepared curry powder, and the onion.
*Information on this ingredient is included in the Glossary.

231

SPICED RICE
Quick and Adventurous

309 calories per serving

Prep Time: 10 minutes
Cook Time: 12–15 minutes

1 Tbsp. vegetable oil
1 tsp. turmeric*
1 tsp. cumin*
1 tsp. ground coriander*
6 cardamon pods,* cracked
1 pinch cinnamon
2 cloves
10 black peppercorns
1 onion, chopped
2$^{1}/_{2}$ cups water or homemade chicken stock
    (see recipe on page 132) or canned nonfat broth
2 Tbsp. raisins
$^{1}/_{2}$ tsp. salt
2 cups rice (basmati or other long grain)

———————————— ❦ ————————————

Heat oil. Saute cardamon, cinnamon, cloves, turmeric, cumin, coriander, and peppercorns for two minutes on low heat. Add onion and $^{1}/_{2}$ cup of water (or stock) and continue cooking for 3 minutes. Add raisins, salt, and the other 2 cups of water (or stock) and the rice. Cover and simmer until rice is tender and liquid is absorbed (12–15 minutes.) This may also be cooked in an automatic rice cooker.

———————————— ❦ ————————————

Serves 4

This is a northern Indian version of rice. It goes exceptionally well with the hot curries called vindaloos.

This rice also makes a great vegetarian meal. Add one cup of cubed veggies such as eggplant and zucchini or a bunch of spinach when you add the rice.

*Information on this ingredient is included in the Glossary.

Vegetables, Pasta, and Risottos

ASPARAGUS BROWN RICE
Easy

211 calories per serving

Prep Time: 30 minutes
Cook Time: 60 minutes

1 cup brown rice, uncooked
2 tsp. walnut or olive oil
$1/2$ onion, chopped
3 cloves garlic, chopped
1 stalk celery, diced
1 bay leaf
1 clove
$1/2$ tsp. poultry seasoning
2 cups homemade low-sodium, nonfat chicken stock
    (see recipe on page 132) or canned nonfat broth
1 cup water
2 Tbsp. parsley, chopped
salt and pepper to taste
16 asparagus spears, steamed for 5–7 minutes,
    and cut into $1^1/2$" pieces
1 Tbsp. lemon juice

Heat oil in a nonstick pan. Add onion, garlic, and celery, and saute until softened, 10–15 minutes. Add rice and saute for 5 minutes more, stirring frequently. Add broth, water, bay leaf, clove, and poultry seasoning. Cover and simmer for 40–50 minutes or until rice is slightly tender. When rice is tender, if there is still liquid in the skillet, remove the cover and continue cooking on higher heat until liquid is gone, about 1–2 minutes. Add parsley and taste for seasoning. Add salt and pepper if necessary.

Toss in asparagus pieces, except for the tips. When serving, arrange the tips on the top of each plate, and add a squeeze of lemon juice just before serving.

Serves 4

This is very good with lemon chicken (see recipe on page 274).

Vegetables, Pasta, and Risottos

FRESH HERB PASTA
Quick and Easy

443 calories per serving

Prep Time: 10 minutes
Cook Time: 10–12 minutes

> 1 lb. pasta (we like farfalle with this recipe). Cook *al dente.** Drain and toss with 1 Tbsp. olive oil.

> 1 or 2 garlic clove(s), mashed
> 3 Tbsp. olive oil
> 2 Tbsp. fresh basil, finely chopped
> 1 Tbsp. fresh tarragon, finely chopped
> 1 Tbsp. fresh thyme, finely chopped
> 2 Tbsp. fresh oregano, finely chopped

———————————————— ❦ ————————————————

Combine garlic and oil and allow to sit while pasta is cooking. Heat garlic and oil in a skillet. Add pasta. Toss until heated through. Remove from heat and toss with herbs. Serve hot or at room temperature.

———————————————— ❦ ————————————————

Serves 4–6

*Information on this term is included in the Glossary.

FRESH VEGETABLE PASTA
Quick and Easy

656 calories per serving
(421 calories in the pasta alone!)

Prep Time: 15 minutes
Cook Time: 15 minutes

8 oz. spaghetti (or pasta of your choice), cooked *al dente**
   and tossed with 2 tsp. olive oil
$1^1/2$ cups homemade nonfat chicken stock
   (see recipe on page 132) or canned nonfat broth
4 tomatoes, chopped
$1/2$ eggplant (about 8 oz.), diced in $1/2$-inch cubes
4 oz. mushrooms, sliced
8 oz. broccoli florets, in small pieces, steamed until just
   cooked, then rinsed with cold water and sprinkled with
   lemon juice to help keep green color
1 to 2 cloves garlic, chopped fine
2 Tbsp. fresh basil, chopped fine
$1/4$ cup white wine
$3/4$ cup water
$1/2$ tsp. sugar
salt and pepper to taste

———————————— ❧ ————————————

Heat a nonstick skillet. Add $1/4$ cup broth. When hot, add mushrooms, eggplant, and garlic, and cook for 4–5 minutes, adding another $1/4$ cup broth as original liquid is absorbed. Add tomatoes. Mix well and add basil, one cup broth, wine, water, salt, pepper, and sugar. Lower heat, cover, and simmer for 5–10 minutes. Remove vegetables with a slotted spoon, and continue cooking remaining liquid on high heat until liquid is reduced by half. Return vegetables to skillet. Add broccoli. Mix and toss with spaghetti.

———————————— ❧ ————————————

Serves 2 as a main dish

*Information on this term is included in the Glossary.

TOMATO SAUCE FOR PASTA
Easy

143 calories per serving

Prep Time: 5 minutes
Cook Time: Several hours or longer

> 3 cloves garlic, chopped
> 1 large onion, chopped
> 1 dried red hot pepper, de-seeded and chopped
> 26 oz. (750 cc) chopped tomatoes (about 2 cups)
> 1 Tbsp. olive oil
> 1¹/₂ cups red wine
> pinch sugar
> ¹/₂ tsp. salt
> black pepper to taste

Saute the garlic, onion, and hot pepper in the oil until slightly browned. Drain off any oil. Add tomatoes, wine, sugar, and salt. Add black pepper to taste. Cook over low heat for several hours (the longer you cook this sauce, the better it becomes), adding some water from time to time if necessary.

Makes about 3 cups or enough for 4 servings of pasta

Vegetables, Pasta, and Risottos

PEARL PASTA WITH MUSHROOMS
Quick and Adventurous

185 calories per serving

Prep Time: 10 minutes
Cook Time: 15 minutes

> 8 oz. pearl pasta (called Israeli Toasted Pasta
>   or Israeli Couscous)
> 8 oz. mixed mushrooms (our favorites for this
>   dish are shiitake*, oyster, and crimini*)
> 4 tsp. olive oil
> 1 onion, chopped
> 2 cloves garlic, chopped
> $^1/_2$ cup water
> $^1/_4$ tsp. salt
> $^1/_8$ tsp. pepper
> 2 Tbsp. parsley, chopped

———————————— ❦ ————————————

Cook the pasta in boiling water for 4 minutes. Turn off the heat and allow it to sit in the pot for another 4 minutes. Drain and rinse. Toss with one teaspoon olive oil.

Heat 3 teaspoons olive oil in a nonstick pan. Add onions and garlic, and cook until onions are transparent, about 3 minutes. Add mushrooms, and continue cooking for 10 minutes. During the cooking, as the pan juices disappear, add a little water as needed. Just before serving, add the pasta and the salt and pepper, and heat through. Sprinkle with chopped parsley.

———————————— ❦ ————————————

Serves 6

*Information on this ingredient is included in the Glossary.

Vegetables, Pasta, and Risottos

VEGETABLE RISOTTO
Quick and Easy

242 calories per serving

Prep Time: 15 minutes
Cook Time: 20–25 minutes

 1 large onion, chopped
 $^1/_2$ cup peas, fresh if possible (out of pods)
 1 cup green beans, fresh if possible, cut into one-inch
    pieces and parboiled for 1–2 minutes
 $^1/_2$ cup (4 oz.) fava beans; if you use them fresh, remove
    from pod, then parboil and remove tough outer skin
 1 cup risotto rice (arborio* or other medium- or
    short-grained rice)
 salt and pepper to taste
 "heat"
 about 2 cups water or stock
 1 Tbsp. oil or 3 Tbsp. vegetable stock (see recipe on page 131)
 1 Tbsp. fresh parsley, chopped

———————————————— ❧ ————————————————

Heat the oil *or* stock in a heavy pot over medium heat. Add onion and cook until translucent, about 3 minutes. Add the rice and cook, stirring for one minute. Now slowly add the water a half cup at a time, stirring constantly. As each half cup is absorbed, add another half cup. Taste the rice occasionally for doneness. When you add the third half cup of water, add the peas, green beans, fava beans, the optional "heat," and salt and pepper. Continue cooking and stirring until rice is *al dente** and mixture is creamy. Serve topped with fresh chopped parsley.

———————————————— ❧ ————————————————

Serves 4

*Information on this term is included in the Glossary.

Vegetables, Pasta, and Risottos

BLACK BEAN RISOTTO
Easy

541 calories per serving
(This may seem high, but remember
that the beans are high in protein and
have almost no fat in this one-dish meal!)

Prep Time: 30 minutes
Cook Time: 20 minutes

1 large onion, chopped
2 cloves garlic, chopped
2 tsp. corn oil
2 cups cooked black beans (homemade or canned)
1 cup risotto rice
water or homemade chicken stock (see recipe on page 132)
chopped green herbs
salt/pepper/lemon juice to taste

Saute onion and garlic in oil until nice and tan. Add rice and mix well. Cook until the rice gets some color. Add a half cup black bean liquid and one cup water or stock. Cook like risotto, adding more water or stock as needed. (Watch out that it doesn't get too thick and turn into dark purple library paste). When rice is *al dente*,* add beans. (**Optional:** One tablespoon tomato paste stirred in thoroughly toward the end of cooking.) Correct seasonings (salt, pepper, lemon juice). Serve garnished with chopped green herbs. (We prefer parsley and thyme.)

Serves 4

*Information on this term is included in the Glossary.

Vegetables, Pasta, and Risottos

SHRIMP RISOTTO WITH RED ONION AND CORN

Quick and Easy

356 calories per serving

Prep Time: 15 minutes
Cook Time: 25 minutes

> 1 lb. shrimp (with shells)
> 1 Tbsp. peanut (or vegetable) oil
> $1/2$ red onion, chopped
> 1 clove garlic, chopped
> 1 pasilla chili,* skinned and chopped
> $1/4$ habanera chili,* minced (**optional:** may also substitute 2 dashes cayenne)
> 1 cup risotto rice (arborio* is usually used; any short-grain rice may be substituted)
> 1 Tbsp. tomato paste
> 6 cups water
> kernels from 1 ear of corn
> $1/8$ tsp. saffron*
> $1/2$ tsp. salt (optional)
> 1 Tbsp. lemon juice
> 1 Tbsp. Parmesan cheese, grated (optional)
> 2 Tbsp. cilantro,* chopped

Shell the shrimp. Add the shells to the water and boil until 4 cups of water remain, about 10 minutes. Strain and save the liquid.

Heat the oil in a pot. Add the onion, garlic, and chilies, and saute until the onion is transparent. Add the rice and mix well. Add tomato paste and stir until absorbed. Add the shrimp liquid, a half cup at a time over moderate high heat, stirring vigorously. Stir until absorbed. Continue adding the shrimp liquid, a half cup at a time, waiting each time for it to become absorbed by the rice. When the rice is slightly firm but not quite done, add the shrimp, saffron, and corn. Stir well. Cook 3–5 minutes longer.

Stir in the lemon juice and the optional salt and Parmesan. Serve hot with cilantro sprinkled on top.

Serves 4

*Information on this ingredient is included in the Glossary.

Vegetables, Pasta, and Risottos

MIDNIGHT RISOTTO
Quick and Easy

387 calories per serving

Prep Time: 15 minutes
Cook Time: 20 minutes

2 shallots, chopped
"heat"
2 tsp. olive oil
$1/2$ lb. shrimp, shelled and cubed
$1/2$ lb. squid, cleaned and sliced
2 cups homemade fish, crustacean, or chicken stock
   (see recipe on pages 130 or 132) or canned nonfat broth
$1^1/2$ cups water
1 cup risotto rice
salt and pepper to taste
Optional: 1 Tbsp. squid ink dissolved in $1/4$ cup water

Heat the olive oil in a pot, and add the shallots. Heat and saute until lightly colored. Add the rice and stir until combined. While cooking, gradually stir in the liquid. (Equal amounts of broth and stock are recommended; however, depending on the concentration of your stock, you will need to balance the flavors to taste.) When the rice is almost completely cooked, add the shrimp and squid, and mix well. Add more liquid as needed to fully cook the rice. Correct the seasonings with salt and pepper, and add the optional squid ink. Serve hot in bowls.

Serves 4

Vegetables, Pasta, and Risottos

LOBSTER AND PEAR RISOTTO

Adventurous

273 calories per serving

Prep Time: 30 minutes
Cook Time: 20 minutes

> 1 small lobster under 1 lb.
> 2 comice pears,* peeled and seeded: one in cubes and
>   one as a puree
> $1/2$ onion, chopped
> $1/2$ serrano chili,* seeded and chopped (or $1/4$ tsp. black pepper)
> $1/2$ cup white wine
> water
> 1 cup lobster stock (don't worry, see below)
> $3/4$ tsp. salt
> 1 cup arborio rice* (or other short- or medium-grained rice)
> 2 cups water
> juice of $1/2$ lemon and more (up to 1 Tbsp.) to taste
> 1 tsp. vanilla extract
> pepper to taste

❦

If you buy a live lobster, steam it. Remove the lobster meat from the shell. Save the drippings and the other substances that are liquid or semi-liquid. Take the tail and the claw meat, and slice in big pieces. Take all of the rest of the lobster (trimmings, leg meat) and lobster drippings, and combine them with the pureed comice pear (seeded, peeled, and pureed with one teaspoon lemon juice). Save.

❦
---

*Information on this ingredient is included in the Glossary.

LOBSTER AND PEAR RISOTTO (cont.)

Remove the gills from the lobster carcass (the things that are sticking up from either side of the head after you take off the carapace*) and throw them away. SAVE THE SHELLS! Use them to prepare the **lobster stock** as follows: Take the lobster shells and the carcass (minus the gills) and chop them up as best you can. Place them into a quart of water, bring to a boil, and then simmer and skim gently for 20 minutes. Strain. You will have less than a quart and probably only about 3 cups. Taste to see what you have made. Remember, it will be diluted and then cooked with rice. Save. This is the lobster broth.

Add the chopped onion and chili to a pot with the wine and a half cup water. Simmer until the mixture is almost dry. Then add a cup of the lobster broth you have made, the lobster pieces, pear puree, and $^3/_4$ tsp. salt. Stir a bit to allow ingredients to blend. Add one cup risotto rice and cook like *risotto* (stir, stir, stir) adding the water as necessary in half-cup portions. (You will probably need about 2 more cups of water.) Add the juice of a half lemon stirred in toward the end. Stir well. Then add the vanilla extract and the lobster pieces and the other comice pear, which has been cubed. Serve hot immediately! Oh, and don't forget to taste for salt, citrus, and pepper, and make the necessary adjustments.

———————————————— ❦ ————————————————

Serves 4

Vegetables, Pasta, and Risottos

SMOKED CHICKEN RISOTTO
Adventurous

345 calories per serving

Prep Time: 15 minutes
Cook Time: 15 minutes

> 1 onion, chopped
> 2 cloves garlic, minced
> 1 tsp. olive oil
> 3 sun-dried tomatoes, chopped
> 1 cup arborio* (or short-grained) rice
> 1 cup smoked chicken, meat only, in chunks ($^1/_2$ smoked chicken)
> $1^1/_2$ cups chopped tomatoes, with juice (fresh or canned)
> 3 Tbsp. flat leaf parsley, chopped
> 1 jalapeno* chili, chopped (optional)
> 4 cups homemade chicken stock (see recipe on page 132) or canned nonfat broth
> extra water as needed
> juice of $^1/_2$ lemon
> salt and pepper to taste

Risotto: In a large pot, heat the oil until its aroma awakens you to action. Add the onion, the garlic, and optional "heat." Saute until onion is lightly browned. Add the sun-dried tomatoes and the rice. Cook for 5 minutes on moderate heat. Add the chicken and cook until well combined, stirring over high heat for 2 minutes. Start adding the stock in one-half to one-cup quantities, stirring after each addition, until the liquid is 80 percent absorbed before you add the next batch. Frequent, hard stirring is one of the tricks to making a good risotto. The rice may require 6 cups of liquid depending on your preparation of the other ingredients. You may add more water as needed. When the rice is done *(al dente)*, add the parsley and mix it well. Add the lemon juice, salt, and pepper. Serve.

Serves 4–6

This is one of our personal favorites. If you stir it well while cooking, it will become creamy without the need to add butter.

*Information on this ingredient is included in the Glossary.

Fish and Shellfish
Main Dishes

Fish and Shellfish Main Dishes

OPEN-FACED CRAB SANDWICHES
Quick and Easy

281 calories per serving

Prep Time: 10 minutes
Cook Time: 8 minutes

> 2 English muffins
> 4 oz. crabmeat
> 1^1/$_2$ Tbsp. catsup or HoMade Chili Sauce (brand name)
> 1 tsp. horseradish
> 1 tsp. Dijon mustard
> ^{1}/$_4$ cup nonfat cottage cheese
> 2 green onions, sliced
> ^{1}/$_2$ stalk celery, chopped
> 1 Tbsp. lemon juice
> 1 Tbsp. parsley, chopped
> salt and pepper to taste
> **Optional:** 1 serrano chili,* chopped

———————————————— ❧ ————————————————

Toast muffin halves until lightly brown. Combine other ingredients and mix well. Spoon onto muffin halves. You may serve them cold or stick them under the broiler until lightly brown. Delicious, low calorie, and filling.

———————————————— ❧ ————————————————

Serves 2

*Information on this ingredient is included in the Glossary.

Fish and Shellfish Main Dishes

SPICY MUSSELS
Quick and Easy

109 calories per serving

Prep Time: 15 minutes
Cook Time: 10 minutes

2 lbs. black mussels, scrubbed and cleaned
"heat"
2 Tbsp. ginger, chopped
2 cloves garlic, sliced
1 onion, chopped
1 tsp. turmeric*
1 Tbsp. coriander powder*
1 tsp. mustard oil* or vegetable oil
1 Tbsp. fish sauce*
handful of cilantro,* chopped
water

In a pot, saute the turmeric and coriander in the oil until nicely browned. Then add the "heat," ginger, garlic, and onion, and mix well. Saute until well combined. Add one cup water and one tablespoon fish sauce. Cook for about 3–4 minutes to combine. You may wish to add 1–2 cups water if too thick. Remember that the mussels will give off liquid when cooked. Add the mussels, stir well, cover, and cook over high heat until the pot boils. Turn off heat and allow the mussels to rest for 1–2 minutes. Ladle into bowls, and sprinkle with cilantro.

Serves 4

*Information on this ingredient is included in the Glossary.

MOROCCAN SHRIMP AND SCALLOPS IN A CHERMOULA NAGE*

Easy

447 calories per serving

Prep Time: 35 minutes
Cook Time: 5 minutes plus rice

$^1/_2$ lb. scallops
$^1/_2$ lb. medium shrimp
1 small onion, grated
$^1/_4$ cup parsley, finely chopped
$^1/_4$ cup cilantro,* finely chopped
"heat"
pinch of salt
1 Tbsp. maple syrup
1 clove garlic, sliced
1 Tbsp. olive oil
3 cups broth or stock
saffron*
4 cups cooked rice

Shell the shrimp and keep the shells. Clean the scallops. Place the shells and the three cups of broth in a pot and simmer for 10 minutes. Strain.

Make the chermoula: Combine the grated onion, saffron, parsley, cilantro, "heat," salt, maple syrup, olive oil, and garlic. Place the shrimp and the scallops into the chermoula mixture, and marinate for 20 minutes.

Combine the warm shrimp broth with the shellfish and the chermoula mix, and simmer until the shrimps and scallops are just tender. Remove the shrimp and scallops and keep warm. Boil the remaining liquid for a few minutes until it gets more concentrated and thickens. Spoon some rice onto the center of a soup plate. Artfully place the shellfish around the rice, and spoon the sauce over all.

Serves 4

Try this without rice, as a delicious soup!

*Information on this term or ingredient is included in the Glossary.

CAJUN DIRTY RICE WITH SHRIMP

Easy

230 calories per serving

Prep Time: 30 minutes
Cook Time: 30 minutes

8–12 medium or large shrimp with shells on
2 cups water
2 cups steamed rice (1 cup uncooked)
1 stalk celery, chopped fine
$^1/_2$ onion, chopped fine
1 clove garlic, chopped fine
$^1/_4$ cup green or red bell pepper, chopped fine
1 tomato, chopped fine
$^1/_2$ cup green onions, green part only, chopped
1 bay leaf
$^1/_2$ tsp. ground thyme
$^1/_4$–$^1/_2$ tsp. cayenne pepper (add $^1/_4$ tsp. first, and taste)
$^1/_2$ tsp. salt
$^1/_2$ tsp. ground white pepper
1 Tbsp. tomato paste
1 Tbsp. peanut (or vegetable) oil
3 Tbsp. parsley, chopped

Heat oil in nonstick skillet. Saute the onion, garlic, bell pepper, celery, tomato, bay leaf, thyme, cayenne, salt, white pepper, and tomato paste. Cook on low heat, stirring occasionally until vegetables are tender, about 15 minutes. While this is cooking, shell the shrimp, and simmer the shells and tails in 2–3 cups water for 10 minutes. Add water as needed. Strain out the shells and save the liquid. When the vegetables are tender, add the shrimp liquid and continue cooking for 5 minutes, stirring occasionally. Slice the shrimp lengthwise, and toss with the rice, green onions, and parsley. Add this mixture to the vegetable mixture, and cook and stir until the shrimp are cooked, about 3-4 minutes.

Serve as a main course or as an accompaniment to Cajun Catfish (see recipe on page 258). Sprinkle with fresh chopped parsley before serving.

Serves 4

CRAB WITH BLACK BEAN SAUCE
Quick and Adventurous

153 calories per serving

Prep Time: 15 minutes
Cook Time: 10 minutes

For 1 Dungeness Crab:
4 green onions, chopped
1 Tbsp. fresh ginger, chopped
2 cloves garlic, chopped
2 Tbsp. sherry
2 Tbsp. white wine
4 Tbsp. water
liquid from crab
$1^1/2$ Tbsp. fermented black beans
a pinch of pepper

This works best with live crab, but you can use precooked crab. After cooking, take the crab apart, and discard the gills and main body shell. Save the liquid from the inside (along with the other semi-liquid parts) and gently precrack the crab so that eating is easier.

In a pot or large saucepan, combine all of the ingredients, including the crab liquid, but not the crab, and heat through. Add more liquid (water), if necessary. Then add the crab and stir. Heat through and serve family style with rice. (**Optional:** One tablespoon cornstarch dissolved in $^1/4$ cup water added toward the end of cooking to thicken the sauce.)

Serves 1–2 per crab

This is a hands-on, fun dish. Have wet towels handy.

GRILLED SHRIMP WITH GINGER TAMARIND RELISH ON A RED PEPPER LAKE

Adventurous

103 calories per serving

Prep Time: 25 minutes
Cook Time: 25 minutes

20 large shrimp with shells
2 cups water
$^1/_2$ lemon
3 red bell peppers

Relish:
$^1/_2$" fresh ginger, julienned
$^1/_4$ red onion, chopped fine
$^1/_2$ fresh red chili, minced
$^1/_2$ bunch cilantro,* chopped
1 tsp. tamarind* concentrate
$^1/_8$ cup rice wine vinegar*
1 stalk lemon grass,* peeled, with white end thinly sliced
1 small tomato, cored, seeded, and diced
$^1/_4$ tsp. sesame oil

Peel the shrimp. Boil the shells in two cups water for about 10 minutes or until the water is reduced to one cup. Strain and save the liquid shrimp stock.

Roast the peppers by placing under a broiler until browned (or blackened) on all sides. Peel, devein, and puree. Combine with the shrimp stock, and cook on low heat for 5 minutes.

Prepare the relish. Dissolve the tamarind in the rice vinegar, and combine with all other relish ingredients. Refrigerate.

Skewer the shrimp to keep them from curling while cooking. Sprinkle with lemon juice and grill for $1^1/2$ minutes on each side or until they turn bright pink. Remove the skewers.

To serve: Place a lake of red pepper puree on a dinner plate. Put a scoop of relish in the center of the plate and surround with grilled shrimp.

Serves 4

This recipe represents a combination of French, American, and Southeast Asian flavors and techniques. The relish is delicious served with many different foods, particularly fish and shellfish.

*Information on this ingredient is included in the Glossary.

251

PAELLA

Adventurous

496 calories per serving

Prep Time: 25 minutes
Cook Time: 40–50 minutes

$^1/_2$ cup white wine combined with $^1/_2$ tsp. powdered
saffron* or 2 Tbsp. saffron threads*
8 large shrimp, shelled
8 mussels
8 littleneck clams
$^1/_2$ cup sliced squid, or 4 scallops
8 oz. lobster tail (or two little ones), cut in quarters
$^1/_2$ lb. halibut or mahi, cut in chunks
1 large onion, chopped
4 cloves garlic, chopped
1 cup tomato, chopped (1 large tomato)
1 green bell pepper, thinly sliced
1 20-oz. jar sliced pimentos
1 bay leaf
4 Tbsp. cilantro*
1 cup frozen peas
3 cups homemade chicken or fish stock
(see recipe on page 130 or 132) or canned
nonfat chicken broth
1 cup arborio rice* (or other short- to medium-grained rice)
salt and pepper to taste
$^1/_2$ orange, thinly sliced

Preheat oven to 375 degrees. Spray an oven-proof pan (or paella pan)
well with vegetable spray and heat. Add onion, garlic, and saute until onion

*Information on this ingredient is included in the Glossary.

PAELLA (CONT.)

is transparent. Add rice and bell pepper, and continue to saute for one more minute. Add wine, saffron mixture, and stir, cooking until the liquid is absorbed. Stir in tomatoes, pimentos, bay leaf, and 3 tablespoons cilantro. Add stock or broth a half cup at a time, stirring, and allowing the liquid to absorb before the next half cup is added. After two cups of broth have been added, put the fish and shellfish into the rice (place the mussels and clams carefully so that they can open freely when they are cooked). Add the final cup of broth, cover, and put in the oven for 12 minutes. Turn off the oven and add the peas. Leave in the oven 4–5 minutes more before serving. Sprinkle with remaining cilantro, salt, and pepper, and decorate with orange slices. Serve.

Serves 6

This makes a wonderful "company" dish with a green salad and a good loaf of bread. The colors are beautiful.

Fish and Shellfish Main Dishes

STEAMED FISH
Quick and Easy

308 calories per serving

Prep Time: 15 minutes
Cook Time: 10 minutes

1 striped bass, about 1^1/$_2$ lbs, cleaned
1 ounce ginger, julienned
5 cloves garlic, sliced
2 hot green chilies, sliced
6 green onions, chopped
4 oz. snap peas
3 cups broth or dashi*
2 Tbsp. rice wine vinegar
"Carrot" for color (yamagobo)*
2 Tbsp. soy sauce
salt

— ❦ —

Rub fish with some salt and let sit for 5 minutes. Then wash fish. Take some of the chopped aromatics and put into the body cavity of the fish. Pour over soy sauce and keep aside for about 15 minutes. In a steamer, place the broth and the rice vinegar. Place the fish on the rack, and steam until almost done (about 10 minutes). Just before the fish is done, add the peas and the rest of the aromatics to the steamer. Cook for a minute or two more. Take the fish out and place on a serving tray, spoon the peas and greens around, and pour some steaming liquid onto the dish. Top with a sprinkling of "carrot" for color. Serve with plain rice.

— ❦ —

Serves 2–4

*Information on this ingredient is included in the Glossary.

FILLET OF SOLE WITH LIME MARINADE
Quick and Easy

174 calories per serving

Prep Time: 5 minutes
Marinate Time: 15 minutes

1 lb. fillet of sole or sand dab

Marinade:
5 Tbsp. fresh lime juice
2 tsp. olive oil
2 Tbsp. honey
$^1/_4$ tsp. pepper
$^1/_4$ tsp. salt

Whisk together all marinade ingredients until well emulsified. Pour over fish and marinate no longer than 15 minutes.

Grill the fish to desired doneness. Serve with couscous (see recipe on page 228).

Serves 4

Fish and Shellfish Main Dishes

POACHED FILLET OF SOLE ON A SPINACH NEST

Quick and Easy

153 calories per serving

Prep Time: 15 minutes
Cook Time: 20 minutes

> 4 sole fillets (if very small, you may need 6 or 8)
> 6 shrimp, chopped
> 6 scallops, chopped
> 1 bunch spinach, well cleaned
> 2 shallots, chopped
> 1 cup white wine
> 1 cup fish stock (or water); the stock can be simply made
>   by boiling the shrimp shells for 15 minutes and straining
> 1 cup water
> lemon juice
> $1/8$ tsp. cayenne (or black pepper)
> salt and pepper to taste
> 4 tsp. red bell pepper or red chili, chopped (optional)

Lightly salt and pepper the fish fillets and lay flat. Cover each with two layers of spinach leaves. Toss the shrimp and scallops together, and place some toward one end of each fish fillet. Roll up each fillet and place seam side down in a baking dish that can go on top of the stove or in the oven. Carefully pour the wine, water, stock, and shallots into the dish to barely cover the fish. Bring to a simmer. Cover with waxed paper and simmer for about 15 minutes, or until fish is white. (You may also poach in a 325-degree oven.) Turn off the heat and allow fish to sit for 5 minutes. Then move the fish very carefully with a slotted spatula to a warm plate. Bring the liquid to a boil and reduce by half. Add the remaining spinach, and cook for 2 minutes.

To serve: Place the spinach on each plate like a nest. Top with fish fillet and a little sauce. Sprinkle bell pepper or red chili over all, and top with a squeeze of lemon juice.

Serves 4

Fish and Shellfish Main Dishes

CURRIED FISH

Easy

201 calories per serving

Prep Time: 15 minutes
Cook Time: 10 minutes

1 lb. fish, firm-fleshed
1 tsp. oil
1 onion
3 green chilies
3 garlic cloves
2 tsp. ginger
1 cup fresh coriander
$1/4$ tsp. cumin seeds*
$1/4$ tsp. fennel seed
1 tsp. coriander powder*
1 tsp. cumin powder*
water
lemon juice

Put the onion, chilies, garlic, ginger, and fresh coriander in a blender, and blend to a paste. In a small amount of oil, fry fish *very briefly* just to get it tan. Take the fish out of the pan. Add the cumin seed and the fennel seed, and roast for a minute or two. Then add the paste and mix well. Simmer for about 5 minutes, adding water if necessary. Add the coriander and cumin powder, and continue to cook for another 5 minutes. Add the fish, a little water, and cook until tender, about 5–8 minutes. Add a squeeze of lemon juice, and serve with plain rice.

Serves 3

*Information on this ingredient is included in the Glossary.

CAJUN CATFISH
Quick and Easy

122 calories per serving

Prep Time: 10 minutes
Cook Time: 5 minutes

1 lb. catfish fillets

Marinade:
$1/4$ tsp. thyme
1 tsp. white ground pepper
$1/8$ tsp. chili powder
$1/8$ tsp. cayenne pepper
1 tsp. onion powder
$1/2$ tsp. garlic powder
1 Tbsp. balsamic vinegar
1 Tbsp. bourbon
salt and pepper to taste

Combine marinade ingredients and rub into and on all surfaces of catfish. Heat a cast-iron skillet until white hot (it will take between 20 and 30 minutes). Quickly dry grill the catfish in the skillet about 2–3 minutes per side until white and tender. Serve with dirty rice (see recipe on page 249).

Serves 4

SHANGHAI CATFISH
Quick and Adventurous

167 calories per serving

Prep Time: 15 minutes
Cook Time: 16–20 minutes

> 2 large catfish fillets
> 1" fresh ginger, julienned
> $1/2$ jalapeno chili,* chopped
> 2 green onions, chopped
> $1/2$ onion, chopped
> 1 tsp. soy sauce
> 1 Tbsp. Chinese oyster sauce*
> $1/2$ red pepper, julienned
> $1/4$ cup Chinese rice wine*
> 1 cup sliced shiitake mushrooms*
> $1/2$ cup homemade fish, chicken, or vegetable stock
>   (see recipes on pages 130–132), or water
> $1/2$ tsp. sesame oil
> 1 Tbsp. peanut oil
> 2 Tbsp. cilantro,* chopped

———————————— ❧ ————————————

Heat the oil in a nonstick pan. Saute the ginger, chili, and onions until slightly golden. Add the soy sauce, oyster sauce, and red bell pepper, and stir well. Add the rice wine, the shiitake mushrooms, and stock (or water). Simmer for 8–10 minutes, stirring occasionally. Remove from pan and keep warm.

Grill the catfish 3–4 minutes on each side. Place on warmed plates. Spoon the sauce over the fish, and sprinkle with cilantro.

———————————— ❧ ————————————

Serves 4

*Information on this ingredient is included in the Glossary.

ROASTED RED SNAPPER WITH GRILLED TOMATILLO SALSA

Quick and Easy

246 calories per serving

Prep Time: 15 minutes
Cook Time: 15 minutes

2 snapper fillets
1 lb. tomatillos* (or green tomatoes)
1 tsp. corn oil
1 clove garlic
Optional: 1 jalapeno chili,* chopped, or $1/4$ tsp. black pepper

1 tsp. corn oil
$1/2$ onion, chopped
$1/2$ cup corn kernels
$1/2$ banana, pureed
1 cup water

Saute whole tomatillos in one teaspoon corn oil until browned, 7–10 minutes. Shake pan frequently while browning so they don't stick. Remove from pan, and pat with paper towel to absorb oil. Cool and puree. Add one clove garlic and the optional jalapeno or black pepper.

Heat one teaspoon oil in a nonstick pan. Saute onion for 3 minutes. Add corn. Continue cooking 3 minutes more. Add tomatillo mixture. Add one cup water and pureed banana, and simmer mixture, stirring occasionally while you cook the snapper.

Roast the snapper for 3 minutes per side or until done.

Pour tomatillo mixture on plate. Add snapper, and sprinkle with chopped cilantro.

Serves 2

Tip: *Watch out when cooking snapper. It's delicate and will break easily if you turn it more than once.*

*Information on this ingredient is included in the glossary

THAI-STYLE SNAPPER
Quick and Adventurous

238 calories per serving

Prep Time: 15 minutes
Cook Time: 15 minutes

> 1 lb. red snapper or four fillets
> 6 green onions, sliced on the diagonal
> 4 cloves garlic, pressed through a garlic press or crushed
> 1 Tbsp. grated fresh ginger
> 2 Tbsp. low-sodium soy sauce
> 1 tsp. sugar or 1 Tbsp. rice wine
> 1 Tbsp. lemon juice
> $^1/_2$ tsp. fish sauce*
> $^1/_4$–$^1/_2$ jalapeno chili* (depending how hot the chili is and
>   how hot you like it) **Optional:** $^1/_2$ tsp. black pepper
> 3 Tbsp. water
> 2 Tbsp. cilantro,* chopped

Spray nonstick pan with vegetable spray. Saute the fish fillets until cooked and browned, about 3 minutes per side. Remove the fish from the pan and keep it warm. Add the green onions and one tablespoon water to the pan and simmer until the onions are soft. Add the garlic, ginger, and 2 tablespoons water, and continue cooking for 2 minutes. Add soy sauce, sugar (or rice wine), lemon juice, fish sauce, and chili (or pepper), and simmer for one minute, stirring occasionally. Spoon the sauce over the fish. Garnish with cilantro and serve.

Serves 4

Delicious and inexpensive.

*Information on this ingredient is included in the Glossary.

BBQ SWORDFISH
Quick and Easy

150 calories per serving

Prep Time: 10 minutes
Cook Time: 6–8 minutes
Marinate Time: 15 minutes

1 lb. swordfish
$^1/_2$ lemon

Marinade:
2 Tbsp. soy sauce
2 cloves garlic, minced
6 Tbsp. green onion, chopped
2 Tbsp. rice vinegar (or 2 Tbsp. white vinegar plus
$^1/_4$ tsp. sugar)
$^1/_4$ tsp. ground ginger
$^1/_4$ tsp. ground pepper

———————————— ❧ ————————————

Combine marinade ingredients. Pour over swordfish, and marinate for 15 minutes. Grill or barbecue swordfish about 3–4 minutes on each side. When grilled, spoon a little marinade on each portion of fish. Top with a squeeze of lemon and serve.

———————————— ❧ ————————————

Serves 4

GRILLED SWORDFISH WITH TOMATO SAUCE
Quick and Easy

154 calories per serving

Prep Time: 15 minutes
Cook Time: 10 minutes

> $1^1/_2$ lbs. swordfish
> 2 bunches spinach, stemmed and washed
> 3 tomatoes, peeled and seeded
> juice of $^1/_2$ lime
> $^1/_2$ tsp. ground black pepper

With an egg-poaching ring or cookie cutter, cut out 6 round pieces of fish. Steam the spinach for 5 minutes. Puree the tomato, and force it through a sieve. Add pepper and lime. Mix well.

Grill the fish about 2-3 minutes on a side or until done. Divide the spinach into 6 parts. Place one part into the ring in the center of a plate. Push down to fill the space. You will have a little disc of spinach about $^1/_4$" high. Put the grilled fish on top. Pour the tomato sauce around the spinach.

Serves 6 as a first course

This is a simple yet elegant dish, with beautiful colors. The fish may be steamed instead of grilled. You can also substitute tuna, shark, or halibut for the swordfish. Or omit the spinach, and sprinkle with chopped basil.

GRILLED FISH WITH MUSSEL SHIITAKE BROTH

Easy and Adventurous

354 calories per serving

Prep Time: 20 minutes
Cook Time: 20 minutes

10 oz. monkfish
2 cups dashi* or fish broth (see recipes on pages 166 and 130)
10 clams, small
2 baby bok choy, chopped
3 large shallots, chopped
4 shiitake mushrooms,* sliced
$1/2$ package enoki mushrooms*, sliced
$1/2$ cup green peas
1 small carrot, julienned (or sliced yamagobo*)
1 Tbsp. rice wine vinegar
$1/4$ cup sake (optional)
$1/8$ tsp. sesame oil
salt and pepper to taste

———————————— ❧ ————————————

Rub the fish with salt, pepper, and a few drops of sesame oil. Save. Make the dashi (**optional:** you can use fish broth). To the dashi or fish broth, add chopped shallots, chopped shiitake mushrooms, chopped bok choy, rice wine vinegar, and a half cup uncooked green peas.

Steam or microwave the clams until they open (about one minute). Save the juice and add to the broth. Shell the clams and save the meat. Simmer the broth while you cook the fish on a grill or pan. When the fish is almost ready, add the sake, clams, and enoki mushrooms to the broth. Cook for a minute or two, divide into two soup bowls, and place a piece of fish on top. Garnish with a carrot or sliced yamagobo.

———————————— ❧ ————————————

Serves 2

*Information on this ingredient is included in the Glossary.

WHITEFISH WITH ORANGE TOMATO SAUCE
Quick and Easy

147 calories per serving

Prep time: 10 minutes
Cook time: 10 minutes

4 whitefish (or Chilean sea bass, mahi mahi, escolar,* or halibut) fillets

Sauce:
1 clove garlic, chopped
2 oranges, peeled (one pureed and one chopped)
1 jalapeno chili,* minced
1/2 tsp. thyme, chopped
1 tsp. oregano, chopped
2 small tomatoes, peeled, seeded, and chopped
1 tsp. coriander seeds*

1 tsp. olive oil
1/8 tsp. salt
1/8 tsp. pepper

lemon juice
2 Tbsp. parsley, chopped

Combine all sauce ingredients in a pot, and simmer, stirring occasionally, while cooking the fish.

Brush the fish with olive oil and salt and pepper, and grill over high heat for about 5 minutes on each side. Make a lake with the sauce on each plate. Place the fish on top. Put a squeeze of lemon juice on each fillet, and sprinkle with parsley just before serving.

Serves 4

Fish and Shellfish Main Dishes

HALIBUT POT AU FEU
Adventurous

317 calories per serving

Prep Time: 30 minutes
Cook Time: 30 minutes

>1 lb. halibut or another white fish
>4 cups homemade nonfat chicken or vegetable stock
>(see recipes on pages 130–131) or canned nonfat broth
>2 carrots, peeled and diced
>4 small boiling potatoes, peeled and diced
>1 leek, white part only, halved and thinly sliced
>$^1/_2$ onion, chopped
>1 clove garlic, chopped
>1 bay leaf
>1 clove
>1 cup white wine
>1 tomato, skinned, seeded, and chopped
>$^1/_2$ tsp. lemon juice
>1 Tbsp. chives, chopped
>3 Tbsp. parsley, chopped
>salt and pepper to taste

———————————————— ❧ ————————————————

In a nonstick pan, saute the onion, leek, and garlic until soft and brown (about 10 minutes), stirring frequently. In a saucepan, bring the broth to a simmer, and add the potatoes, carrots, bay leaf, and clove. When the onion, leek, and garlic are brown, add them to the broth pot. When the carrots and potatoes are tender, remove all the vegetables from the broth. Toss with a little salt and pepper, and keep warm. Add the tomato to the broth. Simmer for one minute. Remove the tomato and set aside. Add wine to the broth, and boil until reduced by half or more. Add a half teaspoon lemon juice,

HALIBUT POT AU FEU (CONT.)

and salt and pepper to taste. If you would like a thicker sauce, use one tablespoon cornstarch dissolved in $1/4$ cup water added to the stock when it has reduced, but is still boiling.

While the sauce is reducing, prepare the fish. Wash and dry it. Sprinkle salt and pepper on both sides. Spray the grill with a vegetable spray before turning on the heat. On medium-high heat, grill the fish about 4 minutes on each side, depending on the thickness of the fish.

To serve: Arrange the vegetables (except tomatoes) in the center of the plate, put the fish on top (sliced or whole), ladle sauce around the vegetables, toss tomatoes over all, and sprinkle with a combined mixture of parsley and chives.

Serves 4

Fish and Shellfish Main Dishes

CHILEAN SEA BASS WITH PAPAYA COULIS AND JICAMA SALSA

Quick and Easy

154 calories per serving

Prep time: 15 minutes
Cook time: 7–8 minutes

1 lb. sea bass

Salsa:
6 ounces jicama,* peeled and diced (about 1 cup)
1/2 red onion, chopped
1/2 bunch cilantro,* chopped
1 Tbsp. lemon juice
1/8 tsp. salt
cayenne or black pepper to taste

Coulis:
1/2 papaya (or mango), pureed (6 Tbsp.)
6 Tbsp. orange juice
1 tsp. lemon juice
1/8 tsp. salt

Combine all ingredients in salsa, and set aside. Combine all ingredients in coulis, and simmer on very low heat for 2 minutes. Blend with a hand mixer. Keep warm.

Grill sea bass for about 3 1/2 minutes on each side or until done.

To serve: place a lake of coulis on the bottom of each plate. Make a nest of jicama salsa in the middle, and top with the fish. (Watch out for bones.) Sprinkle the fish with a squeeze of lemon juice just before serving.

Serves 4

Mmm, mmm, good!

*Information on this ingredient is included in the Glossary.

Fish and Shellfish Main Dishes

GRILLED SALMON WITH JAPANESE SPICES

Quick and Easy

226 calories per serving

Prep Time: 5 minutes
Cook Time: 6-10 minutes
Marinate Time: 15 minutes

2 salmon fillets (or steaks)

Marinade:
2 cloves garlic
$^1/_4$ tsp. dry wasabi* (available in most supermarkets)
1 Tbsp. soy sauce
1 Tbsp. pureed fresh ginger (or $^1/_2$ tsp. dry ginger)
1 Tbsp. lemon juice

— ❧ —

Puree marinade mixture, and rub on both sides of salmon. Marinate for 15 minutes. Scrape off marinade and save. Lightly salt and grill salmon.

— ❧ —

Mix saved marinade with:
1 Tbsp. rice wine and
1 Tbsp. lemon juice

Spoon over the fish.

Top salmon with:
2 Tbsp. green onions, sliced on the diagonal
2 Tbsp. cilantro,* chopped

— ❧ —

Serves 2

*Information on this ingredient is included in the Glossary.

Birds, Game, and Other Low-Fat (Meat) Main Dishes

BASIC RECIPE FOR ROASTED TURKEY OR CHICKEN
Quick and Easy

205 calories per serving

Prep Time: 15 minutes
Cook Time: depends on weight of bird
Marinate Time: 15 minutes or overnight

3-lb. turkey breast, skin removed*

Marinade:
$1/2$ onion
2 cloves garlic
1 Tbsp. parsley
$1/2$ tsp. poultry seasoning
$1/2$ tsp. pepper
1 tsp. salt
1 tsp. paprika (optional)
$1/4$ cup orange juice

———————————— ❧ ————————————

Combine marinade ingredients in a blender or food processor, and puree. Rub well all over turkey. Place turkey into a brown paper bag, and staple shut or wrap tightly in heavy-duty foil. Cook at 350 degrees for 15 minutes per pound, or 45 minutes for this turkey breast. At the end of the cooking time, open bag or foil, and test for doneness with a meat thermometer. Leave the foil or bag open for browning if more cooking is need. When done, remove the bird. Scrape off marinade, and save for gravy, if desired.

———————————— ❧ ————————————

We used turkey breast as an example here, but the recipe will also work well for chicken. This marinade will keep a skinless bird moist while it cooks. Delicious and low fat!

ROASTED TURKEY OR CHICKEN (CONT.)

Gravy/Sauce:
Remaining marinade
Pan juices (remove any fat)
1 cup homemade nonfat chicken stock
    (see recipe on page 132) or canned nonfat broth
$1/2$ cup red wine

———————————————— ❦ ————————————————

Combine above ingredients, and bring to a low boil. Cook 10–15 minutes. Taste for seasoning. You may want to add a little salt and pepper. If you want a thicker sauce, more like a traditional gravy after the sauce has boiled for 10–15 minutes, add one tablespoon cornstarch dissolved in $1/2$ cup cold water. Stir constantly until gravy has thickened. Then remove immediately from heat.

———————————————— ❦ ————————————————

Serves 6

Birds, Game, and Other Low-Fat (Meat) Main Dishes

Birds, Game, and Other Low-Fat (Meat) Main Dishes

LEMON CHICKEN
Easy

187 calories per serving

Prep Time: 15 minutes
Cook Time: 20–25 minutes
Marinate Time: $1/2$ hour

> 4 boneless, skinless chicken breasts
> zest from 2 lemons
> juice from 2 lemons
> 1 Tbsp. Dijon mustard
> 1 tsp. fresh rosemary
> 1 cup homemade nonfat chicken broth
>   (see recipe on page 132) or canned nonfat broth
> salt and pepper to taste
> **Optional:** a dash of cayenne pepper

Remove the zest from two lemons either with a lemon zester or a grater. Set aside. Wash and dry the chicken breasts, and rub with a little salt and pepper. Mix together the juice of two lemons, the Dijon mustard, half the rosemary, and the optional cayenne pepper. Pour over chicken, and marinate for a half hour (no longer).

Remove the chicken from the marinade (save the marinade). Broil, grill, or barbeque the chicken. It will cook quickly because it is boned. Barbequing boneless chicken tends to dry it out, but if you want the flavor, start it on the barbeque (about 5 minutes) to mark and flavor it, then wrap it in foil to finish the cooking.

While the chicken is cooking, combine the chicken broth with 2 tablespoons of the marinade, and boil for 10 minutes. Taste for seasoning. Slice the chicken. Top with cooked marinade and lemon zest. Serve.

Serves 6–8

This dish is very good served with our Asparagus
Brown Rice dish (see recipe on page 233).

LEFTOVER CHICKEN
Quick and Easy, or Adventurous

200 calories per serving

Prep Time 10 minutes
Cook Time: 5 minutes

    5 oz. cooked leftover chicken
    kernels from one ear of corn
    1 leek, chopped
    "heat"
    chicken stock
    $^1/_2$ tsp. oil

———————————— ❧ ————————————

In a nonstick skillet, heat oil, and saute leeks and "heat." Add chicken and enough stock to make a nice gravy. Then add corn, and stir vigorously for a minute or two.

———————————— ❧ ————————————

Serves 2, but can serve 4 if you put it over rice

This recipe lends itself to all kinds of preparations. You can combine just about any vegetable with the chicken; corn is only one option. You can season it Asian, French, Mexican, Thai, or Indian depending on your preference.

Birds, Game, and Other Low-Fat (Meat) Main Dishes

MEDITERRANEAN CHICKEN

Adventurous

215 calories per serving

Prep Time: 30 minutes
Cook Time: 30 minutes to 2 hours

> 6 chicken breasts (bone in)
> 2 cloves garlic, mashed and spread under the skin of the chicken
> 1 Tbsp. olive oil
> $1/4$ cup balsamic vinegar
> 1 onion, chopped
> 4 medium tomatoes, chopped
> 1 red bell pepper, lightly roasted, seeded, and sliced
> 1 green bell pepper, lightly roasted, seeded, and sliced (to roast
>   peppers, simply place under the broiler, turning occasionally,
>   until skin has bubbled and browned. Remove the skin that
>   comes off easily.)
> $1/4$ tsp. ground black pepper
> 1 Tbsp. dry oregano
> 2 to 3 cups water
> $1/2$ cup red wine
> salt to taste
> $3/4$ cup black olives, sliced
> $1/4$ cup parsley, chopped

Heat oil in a heavy pot. Brown the chicken with its skin on. Move the chicken to a plate, and discard the skin. Pour off all but a thin coating of fat from the pan. Add vinegar, and cook until liquid is almost absorbed, scraping up any browned bits from the bottom of the pan.

Add the onions and brown. Then add tomatoes and bell peppers. Cook on low heat, stirring frequently, for 5–7 minutes. Add one cup water, wine, pepper, oregano, olives, parley. Stir until well combined. Return chicken to pot. Taste and add salt if needed. Cover and cook on low heat for 30 minutes (or you may cook as long as two hours if you want the flavor of a chicken stew). Add more water as needed while cooking. The flavor in this dish is enhanced with time, so making it a day ahead will only make it better.

Serves 4–6

Birds, Game, and Other Low-Fat (Meat) Main Dishes

RAYMOND'S GARLIC CHICKEN
Quick and Easy

295 calories per serving

Prep Time: 10 minutes
Cook Time: 20 minutes

4 chicken breasts, boneless and skinless
1 Tbsp. vegetable oil
4 *heads* of garlic, separated into cloves, peeled and
    chopped (if you buy the garlic already peeled and
    chopped, this recipe is really quick)
1 bottle dry white wine
1 cup homemade nonfat chicken stock
    (see recipe on page 132) or canned nonfat broth

In a nonstick pan, brown the chicken in one teaspoon oil and remove. In the same skillet, saute the garlic in 2 teaspoons of the oil, stirring constantly, until it looks like dry buckwheat kernels (nicely browned). Add the wine and stock. Stir and boil off the alcohol, about 5 minutes. Add the chicken, and simmer for about 15 minutes. Remove the chicken and keep warm. Strain the liquid, reserving the garlic. Reduce the liquid until thick.

Serve over chicken, and accompany with a small mound of garlic bits on the side.

Serves 4

*This is a variation of a classic French dish, but without any cream to thicken the sauce. Most people will not guess that it is made with **sooo** much garlic. If you cook the garlic until just before it burns, it will be perfect.*

Birds, Game, and Other Low-Fat (Meat) Main Dishes

CHICKEN BALI-H'AI
Quick and Adventurous

204 calories per serving

Prep Time: 10 minutes
Cook Time: 20 minutes
Marinate Time: 2 hours minimum

3 chicken breasts, skinned and cut into pieces
$^1/_2$ cup homemade nonfat chicken stock
   (see recipe on page 132) or canned nonfat broth
$^1/_2$ cup orange juice
salt and pepper to taste

Marinade:
1 dried red chili, crumbled
1 onion, chopped
2 cloves garlic, minced
2 tsp. shrimp paste*
$^1/_2$ tsp. tomato paste
1 Tbsp. peanut oil
1 Tbsp. brown sugar
2 Tbsp. rice wine vinegar

Prepare the marinade: Saute the chilies, onion, shrimp paste, and garlic in the peanut oil until the onion is soft, about 3 minutes. Add the sugar, and saute until the onion turns brown, about 3 minutes. Add the tomato paste and rice wine vinegar, and simmer 20 minutes. LET THE MARINADE COOL, then add the chicken and marinate for a couple of hours or overnight in the refrigerator.

Take the chicken out of the marinade, and saute it in batches. Put the

*Information on this ingredient is included in the Glossary.

CHICKEN BALI-H'AI (cont.)

chicken aside, and add any remaining marinade and cook until browned. Pour off the oil and loosen the brown bits by adding chicken broth and the orange juice and scraping the pan. Return the chicken back to the pot, stir, correct the seasoning, and simmer for about 5–10 minutes. Add more water or broth if necessary. There should be a little sauce at the end of cooking. Serve with rice.

Serves 4

This is a delicious dish with many intricate flavors. Don't be put off by the initial smell of the shrimp paste. It adds a complexity that will expand the flavors of the food.

Birds, Game, and Other Low-Fat (Meat) Main Dishes

CAJUN CREOLE CHILI

Adventurous

385 calories per serving

Prep Time: 30 minutes
Cook Time: 1^1/$_2$ hours

> 1 smoked ham hock
> 3 cups homemade nonfat chicken stock
>   (see recipe on page 132) or canned nonfat broth
> 3 cups water
> 1 lb. chicken, boned, skinned, and cubed
> 2 links hot Cajun duck sausage, sliced
> 2 garlic cloves, minced
> ^{1}/$_8$ tsp. cayenne pepper
> ^{1}/$_2$ lb. beans (pinto or kidney)
> 1 onion, chopped
> 1 green bell pepper, seeded and chopped
> 3 stalks celery, chopped
> 3 cloves garlic, chopped
> 1 jalapeno* chili, chopped
> 2 tsp. vegetable oil
> 1 Tbsp. flour

Mix the chicken and sausage with 2 cloves garlic and cayenne. Soak the beans in water overnight or bring 4 cups of water to a boil. Add the beans, and turn off the heat. Let the beans rest in the water for one hour. Drain. Saute the chicken and sausage in hot oil until browned. Remove with a slotted spoon and drain. Pour off almost all of the oil and add the flour. Stir, watching that it does not burn. Add all the rest of the ingredients except garlic and beans. Cook 5 minutes. Mix well, scraping the bottom of the pan. Add the beans with the ham hock, chicken stock, and water, and cook until beans are tender (about one hour) and the sauce is reduced and thick.

Serves 6

*Information on this ingredient is included in the Glossary.

ROASTED HENS
Quick and Easy

703 calories per serving (with skin left on)

Prep Time: 15 minutes
Cook Time: 30–40 minutes
Marinate Time: $1/2$–4 hours

> 4 Cornish game hens
> 1 bunch parsley
> 1 bunch tarragon
> 1 bunch thyme
> 1 sprig rosemary
> 1 bunch chervil*
> 6 cloves garlic, chopped
> 2 Tbsp. olive oil
> 1 Tbsp. lemon juice
> salt and pepper

("Bunch" is the amount of the herb you get in your store if you buy "one." We assume that the bunch of tarragon is much smaller than the bunch of parsley.)

Chop the herbs coarsely. Add garlic, salt, and pepper, and mix well. Clean the birds and stuff them with the herb mixture. Rub them with oil and lemon juice, and sprinkle with salt and pepper. Place the birds in a plastic beg with any leftover herbs. Place in the refrigerator to marinate from a half hour to four hours.

When you are ready, place the hens on a spit and roast for 20–40 minutes (depending on the heat of your rotisserie). **Option:** roast in a 350-degree oven for 40 minutes, or until the juice is clear (not bloody) when the hen is pierced between the thigh and the body. Cut the birds in half before serving. The herbs should be removed from the birds and placed on the plate for color when serving.

Serves 4–8

These birds are bursting with herb aroma. They are delightful served on a roasted red pepper sauce (see recipe on page 314) with garlic mashed potatoes.

*Information on this ingredient is included in the Glossary.

Birds, Game, and Other Low-Fat (Meat) Main Dishes

POUSSIN (OR CHICKEN) CASSOULET

Adventurous

400 calories per serving

Prep Time: 20 minutes
Cook Time: 35 minutes

> 1 turkey Cajun sausage
> 1 poussin* (chicken, or other small bird)
> 1 onion, chopped
> 4 cloves garlic, chopped
> 1 cup lentils
> 1 tsp. coriander* seed
> 1 Tbsp. parsley chopped
> 2 tsp. olive oil
> salt/pepper/lemon juice to taste
> water

Slice the sausage. Put it into a shallow pan with some water to cover and cook *until all of the water has evaporated.* Then let the sausage cook in whatever fat has been rendered until brown. Take out the sausage and drain on paper towels. Pour off any remaining fat from the pan and add a half cup water. Scrape up all of the bits in the pan and bubble for a few minutes to get everything combined. Then pour the liquid into a bowl and add the cut-up sausage. Cover and save.

Take one poussin (actually you can use any small bird or part thereof, such as quail, Cornish hen, or chicken breast or leg). Cut up the bird and sprinkle with salt and pepper and some oil. Saute in a nonstick pan until half done. Remove meat from the pan, and take the meat and skin off the bones. Save the bones for another time for preparing broth or stock. Discard the skin.

*Information on this ingredient or term is included in the Glossary.

POUSSIN (OR CHICKEN) CASSOULET (CONT.)

Saute onion and garlic in oil. When slightly brown, add one cup of lentils, the chopped-up sausage, and about 5 cups of water. (At this point, turn on your oven to 450 degrees.) Cook until the lentils are soft, adding more water as necessary. Taste for seasoning, adding salt, pepper, and/or citrus as necessary. When the lentils are done, puree or mash about $^1/_4$ of the lentils and stir well. Add the coriander seed. The lentils should be slightly "runny." Add more water if necessary. Taste again and correct seasoning. Divide the lentils into two (or four) oven-proof ramekins,* and put the poussin meat over the lentils, slightly pushing them into the legume. Place the ramekins in the oven for about 5 minutes until they start to bubble. Take them out, sprinkle with parsley, and serve in the ramekin. (Consider a burst of fresh herbs sprinkled on top before serving.)

Serves at least 2; can be stretched to 4

GRILLED MARINATED QUAIL

Quick and Easy

300 calories per serving

Prep Time: 10 minutes plus time to marinate
Cook Time: 5 minutes

2 quail
salt and pepper to taste

Marinade:
5 cloves garlic, peeled
1 small onion, peeled and chopped
2 Tbsp. homemade chicken stock (see recipe on page 132)
     or canned nonfat broth
1 Tbsp. white wine
3 Tbsp. olive oil
2 tsp. red wine vinegar

―――――――――――――――――― ❧ ――――――――――――――――――

Place all of the marinade ingredients in a blender and puree until smooth. Place the quail in the marinade, and cover and marinate for as long as possible (up to 24 hours).

When ready to cook, heat the grill, take the birds out of the marinade, and sprinkle them with a pinch of salt and black pepper. Grill until tender (just a few minutes) and serve hot.

―――――――――――――――――― ❧ ――――――――――――――――――

Serves 2

GRILLED MARINATED QUAIL II
Quick and Adventurous

284 calories per serving

Prep Time: 10 minutes plus time to marinate
Cook Time: 5 minutes

2 quail
salt and pepper to taste

Marinade:
1 Tbsp. olive oil
1 large garlic clove
1 tsp. coriander powder*
1 tsp. cumin powder*
1 tsp. hot paprika
2 Tbsp. cilantro*, chopped

Place all of the marinade ingredients in a blender, and puree until smooth. Place the quail in the marinade, cover, and marinate for as long as possible (up to 24 hours).

When ready to cook, heat the grill, take the birds out of the marinade, and sprinkle them with a pinch of salt and black pepper. Grill until tender (just a few minutes) and serve hot.

Serves 2

*Information on this ingredient is included in the Glossary

DUCK BREASTS STUFFED WITH COUSCOUS ROASTED WITH A CHERMOULA COAT AND SERVED ON A LAKE OF LEMON SAUCE WITH PRESERVED FRUIT

Adventurous

507 calories per serving

Prep Time: 30 minutes
Cook Time: 30 minutes

Chermoula (see recipe on page 316)
5 oz. medium couscous* (about $^3/_4$ cup)
2 cups boiling water
4 shallots, chopped
1 Tbsp. olive oil
1 cup mixed dried fruits, chopped
2 duck breasts (preferably Maigret or Muscovy)
    (about 1 lb. meat each)
6 Tbsp. homemade chicken stock
    (see recipe on page 132) or canned nonfat broth
3 Tbsp. lemon juice
$^1/_2$ cup white wine
$^1/_2$ cup water
1 bay leaf
3" cinnamon stick
1 tsp. oil
salt and pepper to taste
2 Tbsp. parsley, chopped

---

*Information on this ingredient is included in the Glossary.

DUCK BREASTS ... (CONT.)

Prepare the Chermoula (on page 316), and puree it in a blender. You will have about a half cup.

"Cook" the couscous. Spread 5 oz. ($^3/4$ cup) evenly on a sheet pan or in a bowl and add 2 cups boiling water. Stir now and then until the pasta is soft. Meanwhile, saute the 4 chopped shallots in a little oil in a nonstick pan. They must brown but not get black. Add the shallots to the couscous, and season to taste with salt and pepper and "heat."

Prepare the sauce: Heat the cup of mixed fruit, the 6 tablespoons chicken broth, the 3 tablespoons lemon juice, a half cup white wine, a half cup water, 1 bay leaf, and 3" cinnamon stick, and simmer for 20 minutes or more until the flavors are well combined. Take out the cinnamon and bay leaf.

Prepare the duck breasts: Skin and clean them, removing the thick outer layer of fat. (It would be best at this point to rub them with some of the Chermoula and let them rest for an hour or all day in the refrigerator.) When you are ready to begin the actual cooking: In the center of the breast on one side (*the narrow side*), make a small slit and put in a knife and cut in the middle of the breast to form a cavity (sort of like a pita pocket). Take the couscous and place it in a pastry bag, OR put it into the breast with a spoon. In either case, fill the cavity you have created with the couscous mixture. Rub with more Chermoula. Cook on a grill until the duck breast is done. It won't take too long, depending on the heat. Serve when heated through and the duck is crisp on the outside and rosy, but not bloody, underneath.

To serve: Slice the breasts in the short direction, about one inch thick, about three slices per plate, artfully arranged. Then pour the sauce *around* (not over) the duck, and sprinkle some parsley over the dish.

Serves 4

This recipe is a lot of fun and presents very nicely.

OSTRICH MEAT LOAF WITH CORN ADOBO
Quick and Easy

334 calories per serving

Prep Time: 15 minutes
Cook Time 15–20 minutes

    10 oz. ostrich* meat, ground

Adobo:
5 pasilla chilies,* dried
1 cup cooked corn kernels
$1/3$ cup homemade chicken stock (see recipe on page 132)
    or canned nonfat broth
2 Tbsp. shallots, chopped
1 Tbsp. lemon juice

1 cup cooked corn kernels
$1/2$ onion, chopped
1 clove garlic, chopped
1 beaten egg white (optional)
1 tsp. oil
1 cup broth
chopped parsley for garnish

Preheat oven to 400 degrees.

———————————— ❧ ————————————

Prepare the adobo: First soak the chilies until they are soft (about 10 minutes). Puree them with the broth, the chopped shallots, and the lemon juice. Mix in the corn kernels, and set aside to let it season up. Taste and correct seasoning (adding salt and pepper and lemon juice as needed).

OSTRICH MEAT LOAF (CONT.)

Prepare the ostrich: Combine the ostrich meat, 2 Tbsp. (or more) of the adobo, and the corn. Saute the onion and garlic in one teaspoon oil in a nonstick pan until browned. Cool and then combine with the meat. Mix well and add one beaten egg white (optional). Salt and pepper to taste.

Spoon the mixture into 2 ramekins* and place in the oven until bubbling. Combine the rest of the adobo with the stock, heat through, and correct the seasonings. Turn the loaf out of the ramekin and put it on a plate, spoon the adobo around, and sprinkle with some chopped parsley.

— ✿ —

Serves 2 main portions

*Information on this ingredient or term is included in the Glossary.

Birds, Game, and Other Low-Fat (Meat) Main Dishes

TRADITIONAL MEATLOAF MADE WITH OSTRICH
Quick and Adventurous

157 calories per serving

Prep Time: 15 minutes
Cook Time: 30 minutes

1 lb. ground ostrich*
1 onion, chopped fine
1 clove garlic, minced
1 tsp. Worcestershire
1 tsp. dried oregano
2 Tbsp. parsley, chopped
$1/2$ cup canned tomatoes, chopped
1 egg white
$1/2$ tsp. salt or less
$1/4$ tsp. pepper or less

Preheat oven to 350 degrees. Combine all ingredients. Form into loaf, and bake 30 minutes or until done.

Serves 4

In the Dark Ages, when I used to make meatloaf out of beef and pork, I was constantly removing fat from the loaf pan as my meatloaf cooked. You will be amazed at how little fat is produced from this meat.

*Information on this ingredient is included in the Glossary.

OSTRICH BOLOGNESE
Quick and Easy

322 calories per serving

Prep Time: 10 minutes
Cook Time: 30 minutes (or all day if you make it in your crockpot)

 $^3/_4$ lb. ground ostrich*
 2 tsp. fresh thyme, chopped
 1 onion, chopped
 4 cloves garlic, chopped
 2 red dried chilies, de-seeded
 $^1/_2$ cup cognac, or brandy, Calvados, Armagnac, or any
   nonsweet eau de vie
 $1^1/_2$ cups tomato puree
 2 cups water
 2 cups red wine
 $^1/_4$ tsp. salt
 $^1/_4$ tsp. ground black pepper
 2 Tbsp. tomato paste
 2 Tbsp. parsley, chopped

Saute the $^3/_4$ pound ostrich, the 2 teaspoons thyme, one chopped onion, 4 chopped garlic cloves, and 2 red dried chilies, de-seeded and torn apart (wear gloves or wash immediately after) in some olive oil (don't worry, most of it's coming out after it has done its job). When everything is nice and tan to mahogany in color, add the cognac and ignite it with a match (or by turning the pan over so that the flame of the stove hits the top of the pot). When the flame dies out, add the 2 cups water and the 2 cups red wine. Watch until they come to a boil (so the alcohol is gone), and then simmer and skim, skim, skim. When the top of the simmering pot does not have any more oil or other blemishes on its surface, you may add the $1^1/_2$ cups tomato puree, the 2 tablespoons tomato paste, and the 2 tablespoons chopped parsley. Cook for a half hour to 2 hours, or put this in your crockpot with the other ingredients and cook according to your manufacturer's instructions.

Serve with pasta.

Serves 4

*Information on this ingredient is included in the Glossary.

Birds, Game, and Other Low-Fat (Meat) Main Dishes

OSTRICH OYSTER STEAK WITH PUMPKIN / MANGO ADOBO
Adventurous

252 calories per serving

Prep Time: 30 minutes
Cook Time: 15 minutes

Make the adobo:
6 dried chili pasilla*
1 onion, chopped
4 cloves garlic, chopped
1 Tbsp. peanut oil
$1/2$ cup pumpkin seed powder
$1/2$" cinnamon
3 whole cloves
$1/4$ tsp. dried thyme
1 chili chipotle*
1 tsp. sugar
$2/3$ cup pureed mango

chopped parsley or cilantro

Toast the chilies and soak them in water to cover. In the oil, saute the onion, garlic, cinnamon, cloves, thyme, and pumpkin seed powder until nicely browned. Place on paper towel to remove remaining oil. Add the cooked mixture to a blender. Remove the pasilla chilies from their soaking liquid, and remove the seeds and discard. Add the chilies and the soaking liquid to the blender, as well as all of the other ingredients. Puree well. Place in a pan and cook slowly for 10 minutes, strain, and keep warm. Correct the seasoning with salt and pepper.

*Information on this ingredient is included in the Glossary.

OSTRICH OYSTER STEAK (CONT.)

❧

1 ostrich oyster steak butterflied into two pieces (about $^3/4$ lb.)
5 cloves garlic
$^1/_2$ tsp. oregano
1 tsp. peanut oil

❧

Grind garlic, oregano, and peanut oil to a paste, and coat the ostrich. Let it marinate for a half hour or more. Grill the ostrich to desired doneness. Slice, and artfully place on a plate with the adobo. Garnish with chopped parsley or cilantro.

❧

Serves 4 as a main course

Birds, Game, and Other Low-Fat (Meat) Main Dishes

ROASTED OSTRICH IN A CHIPOTLE MARINADE

Adventurous

375 calories per serving

Prep Time: 1 hour
Cook Time: 20 minutes

1 lb. ostrich meat (with all fat removed)
1 Tbsp. oregano
2 cloves garlic, crushed
2 tsp. olive oil
"heat"
5 dried pasilla chilies,* seeded
2 chipotle* chilies
1 onion, chopped
1 carrot, chopped
$^{1}/_{4}$ cup brandy
$^{1}/_{4}$ cup balsamic vinegar
2 cups homemade chicken stock
    (see recipe on page 132) or canned nonfat broth
1 Tbsp. sun-dried tomato paste
    (you can also use regular tomato paste)
2 Tbsp. parsley, chopped
1 cup water

Rub the ostrich with the oregano, garlic, one teaspoon olive oil, and "heat." Cover and set aside in a cool area. Dry-roast the pasilla chilies. Saute the onion and carrot in one teaspoon olive oil. When the vegetables are tan, combine them with both types of chilies, and puree in a blender with $^{1}/_{4}$ cup balsamic vinegar plus one cup water. Place the puree in a saucepan, cook until caramelized, then flame with the brandy. Add 2 cups of broth or water, stir well, and correct the seasonings.

Roast the ostrich, basting with some of the sauce from time to time. When cooked to desired state, slice the venison, put on a dish, and surround with the sauce. Sprinkle on the parsley, and serve hot.

Serves 4

*Information on this ingredient is included in the Glossary.

ROASTED VENISON ON A RED WINE MIRAPOIX

Adventurous

375 calories per serving

Prep Time: 30 minutes
Cook Time: 60 minutes
Marinate Time: 1–10 hours

     1 lb. venison, trimmed of all fat
     2 shallots, minced
     1 tsp. fresh thyme, chopped
     2 Tbsp. Armagnac or Cognac

Sauce:
     1 Tbsp. olive oil
     2 carrots, chopped
     1 leek, white part only, chopped
     2 stalks celery, chopped
     1 onion, chopped
     1½ cups homemade nonfat chicken stock
        (see recipe on page 132) or canned nonfat broth
     1½ cups red wine
     1 cup water
     1 bay leaf
     2 whole cloves
     salt and pepper to taste
     2 Tbsp. parsley, chopped

Rub the venison with the shallots, thyme, and Armagnac or Cognac. Marinate 1–10 hours. Remove the venison from the marinade, and save the liquid. In a large pot, heat the oil. Add the carrots, celery, onions, and leek, and cook, stirring frequently for 20 minutes. Remove this mixture from the pot and puree. To the same pot, add the chicken broth, wine, water, marinade liquid, bay leaf, and cloves. Scrape up any pieces from the bottom of the pot. Simmer 15 minutes. Add the pureed vegetable, and continue simmering, stirring frequently for 15 minutes more. Grill the venison on high heat until cooked to your liking. (We like to serve venison medium rare.) Place 2–4 tablespoons of pureed sauce in the middle of each plate. Slice the venison and arrange on top of the pureed vegetables. Top with chopped parsley and serve.

ROASTED VENISON WITH BALSAMIC SYRUP

Easy

447 calories per serving

Prep Time: 10 minutes
Cook Time: 30 minutes

> 1 lb. venison (chops will be fine)
> 8 shallots, chopped
> 3 ribs celery, chopped
> 2 carrots, chopped
> bay leaf
> 1 clove
> 1 Tbsp. olive oil
> 8 cups water (if using bones and trimmings) *or*
>   8 cups homemade beef stock or canned nonfat broth
> 1 cup balsamic vinegar

Meticulously clean the venison of all fat and bones. Sprinkle with pepper and save. (If you are making stock from scratch, chop and brown the bones and trimmings. In a pot, saute the shallots, celery, and carrots in some olive oil until nicely colored. Add the bones and trimmings, bay leaf, one clove, and water. Bring to a simmer, and skim off all of the fat and scum that rises to the surface. Simmer slowly until reduced to about half the volume, and strain.) In a small pot, boil the balsamic vinegar to about $1/3$ cup or less (it should be thick like molasses), and then stir in the reduced stock. (If you're not making your own stock, reduce store-bought stock by boiling, and add the balsamic vinegar to it.) Simmer and correct the seasonings. The syrup should be slightly thick, sweet, and a bit tart. Keep warm.

Saute, roast, or grill the venison. Serve with some creamy polenta (see recipe on page 230), and surround with the sauce.

Serves 2–4

GRILLED LAMB WITH LEEK SAUCE
Adventurous

383 calories per serving

Prep Time: 30 minutes
Cook Time: 10 minutes

Please note: Although we have mentioned that lamb has a higher fat content than most low-fat meats, if you trim it well and have a lean cut, it's okay every once in a while.

        1 rack of lamb: about 8 ribs (meticulously cleaned of all
            fat and bones, leaving about 9 oz. lean meat)
        3 large leeks, cleaned and chopped
        3 shallots, chopped
        $1/4$ cup brandy
        2 Tbsp. lemon peel
        6 cups water
        $1/8$ tsp. lemon juice
        3 green onions, sliced

———————————— ❧ ————————————

Take all of the scraps of the lamb (but not the fat) and the bones, and chop them up. Saute in a saucepan over high heat until everything is brown. Remove the solids and save. Pour off all of the oil, but don't wipe the pan. Add the leeks and shallots, and saute until tan. Add back the lamb bones and trimmings. Mix well and add the brandy. Flame. When the flame goes out in the pan, add the lemon peel and 6 cups water, and simmer for at least 20 minutes. Skim the sauce frequently. You will end up with less than a cup of fairly thick sauce. Correct the seasoning with lemon juice and pepper. Save.

Grill the lamb until perfect (about 5 minutes). Slice. Place some sauce on a plate, and top with the meat. Sprinkle green onions over the dish and serve.

———————————— ❧ ————————————

Makes enough for 3 main courses or 4 appetizers

Birds, Game, and Other Low-Fat (Meat) Main Dishes

LAMB SHASHLIK
Quick and Easy

189 calories per serving

Prep Time: 15 minutes
Cook Time: 10–15 minutes
Marinate Time: ¹/₂ hour–2 hours

Please note: Although we have mentioned that lamb has a higher fat content than most low-fat meats, if you trim it well and have a lean cut, it's okay every once in a while.

> 16 oz. lamb tenderloin, all fat removed
> 1 onion, chopped
> 4 cloves garlic, chopped
> ¹/₂ cup red wine vinegar
> ¹/₂ cup water
> ¹/₄ tsp. ground cloves
> ¹/₄ tsp. ground cinnamon
> ¹/₄ tsp. ground pepper
> ¹/₂ cup red wine
> 1 Tbsp. mint, finely chopped

Combine vinegar, water, ground cloves, cinnamon, and pepper in a saucepan. Boil for 2 minutes. Cool. Add red wine. Add onions and garlic, and puree. Pour over lamb, and marinate for a half hour to 2 hours. Remove the lamb.

Broil or roast the lamb, turning so that all sides are browned. Salt to taste.

Return the marinade to the saucepan and boil for 5–10 minutes until it has reduced in volume to about a half cup. This may be used as a sauce for the lamb. Sprinkle with chopped mint.

Serves 4

GRILLED VEAL CUTLET WITH MANGO SAUCE

Adventurous

555 calories per serving

Prep Time: 30 minutes
Cook Time: 1 hour

Two veal chops, with bone
1 Tbsp. oil
1 onion, chopped
2 carrots, chopped
2 ribs celery, chopped
3 sprigs thyme
2 cups dry white or red wine
2 cups homemade chicken stock (see recipe on page 132)
    or canned nonfat broth
1 Tbsp. lemon juice
1 mango, peeled and pureed
1 Tbsp. thyme or parsley, chopped

❧

Cut the chops from the bone. Trim the meat, and save all of the scraps, including the fat. Take a heavy cleaver, and splinter the bones into small pieces. Heat the oil in a stockpot and add the bones. Stir occasionally until brown. Then add the meat and scraps. Lower the heat, and saute the mixture until the meat colors a dark tan. Pour off all of the fat. Add the onion, carrots, celery, and thyme to the pot. Stir well. When the onion begins to color, add the wine and boil off the alcohol. Add two cups chicken broth, and simmer the mixture for as long as possible (at least an hour over low heat). Skim the sauce frequently to remove any scum and fat that rises to the top. Add the lemon juice, and continue cooking until you have about 2 cups. Strain the liquid and discard the solids. You will end up with about one cup of stock. Puree the mango and add it to the stock. Simmer for about 10 minutes. The sauce should be thick, but still liquid. Taste for salt and pepper, and add if necessary. Sprinkle the veal with one teaspoon oil and a pinch salt and pepper. Grill over a hot fire until done to your liking (probably about 5 minutes). Place some of the mango sauce on a plate, and put the meat on top. Sprinkle with parsley or thyme for color.

❧

Serves 2

A little higher in fat, so save for an occasional treat.

GRILLED PORK TENDERLOIN MARINATED ASIAN STYLE
Quick and Adventurous

323 calories per serving

Prep Time: 15 minutes
Cook Time: 15 minutes
Marinate Time: ½ hour–4 hours

1 lb. pork tenderloin (all fat removed)

Marinade:
4 cloves garlic, pressed through a garlic press or crushed
2 Tbsp ginger, chopped
1 mango, diced
1 Tbsp sesame oil
2 dried red chilies, crushed (or 1 tsp. ground black pepper)
½ cup rice wine
¼ cup rice wine vinegar*
1 Tbsp. Chinese bean sauce
½ Tbsp. oyster sauce*
3 Tbsp. cilantro,* chopped
4 green onions, slivered
1 Tbsp. lemon juice
soy sauce to taste (you may not need any)
1 Tbsp. Hoisin sauce (optional)

Combine all the above ingredients (except for one green onion and the lemon juice), and marinate the pork in this mixture for at least 30 minutes but no more than 4 hours. Separate marinade and pork. Grill the pork for about 6 minutes on each side. While it is grilling, add lemon juice to the marinade and boil for 5 minutes. To serve, slice the pork on the diagonal. Spoon the marinade over or around the pork. If you prefer a thicker sauce, add a cornstarch and water mixture. Garnish with the last slivered green onion.

Serves 4

This dish is really very easy. It's great for company and always gets raves.

*Information on this ingredient is included in the Glossary.

Sweets

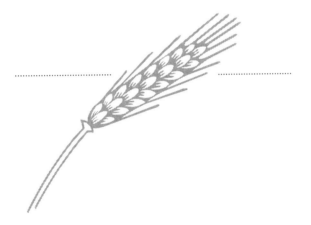

STRAWBERRY MANGO SORBET

Quick and Easy

76 calories per serving

Prep Time: 10 minutes
Cook Time: 30 minutes

> 1 cup simple syrup (see recipe below)
> $^1/_2$ cup juice from a jar of mangoes
> 1 cup strawberry puree (about 2 baskets of strawberries)
> $^1/_2$ cup mango puree (about $^1/_2$ mango)
> 1 egg white
> 1 Tbsp. lemon juice

Combine the simple syrup, lemon juice, mango juice, and the fruit purees. Beat the egg white until stiff and fold into the fruit mixture. Freeze in a sorbet maker or an ice cream freezer.

Serves 6

SIMPLE SYRUP

Quick and Easy

96 calories per serving

Prep Time: 1 minute
Cook Time: 5 minutes

> 4 cups sugar
> 4 cups water

Combine and cook, stirring over low heat for 5 minutes. Cool and refrigerate for later use.

This syrup is used as a base for all fruit sorbets.

PUMPKIN RAISIN SORBET
Quick and Easy

92 calories per serving

Prep Time: 10 minutes
Cook Time: 20 minutes

1 cup simple syrup (see recipe on previous page)
$1/2$ cup water
$3/4$ cup canned pumpkin, pureed
$1/8$ tsp. ground ginger
$1/4$ cup raisins
$1/4$ cup bourbon
2 Tbsp. lemon juice
1 Tbsp. grated lemon peel
1 egg white

Combine the simple syrup with the water. Boil for one minute. Cool. Combine the bourbon and raisins. Plump the raisins by heating in the microwave for one minute or on the stove in boiling water for 3 minutes. Beat egg white until stiff. Fold in all other ingredients. Freeze in a sorbet maker or an ice cream maker.

Serves 6–8

Sweets

BANANA TAMARIND SORBET WITH STRAWBERRY TIPS ON STRAWBERRY PUREE

Quick and Adventurous

101 calories per serving

Prep Time: 20 minutes
Freeze Time: 30 minutes

> 2 baskets strawberries
> 3 bananas, pureed (1²/₃ cup puree)
> 4 Tbsp. tamarind* concentrate
> 4 Tbsp. lemon juice
> 3 Tbsp. water
> 1 cup simple syrup (see recipe on page 302)
> 1 Tbsp. mint, finely chopped

Clean the strawberries and remove the stems. Cut the tips off (¹/₂" from bottom) and save for decorating the plate. Puree the remaining strawberry parts, and strain to remove seeds.

Mix tamarind concentrate, lemon juice, and water until the tamarind is well incorporated. Combine with the banana puree, simple syrup, and mint.

Freeze in a sorbet maker or an ice cream freezer.

To serve: Place a spoonful or two of sorbet on each plate. Surround with strawberry puree, and decorate with strawberry tips.

Serves 6

In addition to tasting good, this sorbet is fun because it looks like chocolate ice cream. You'll have your guests guessing what the ingredients are.

*Information on this ingredient is included in the Glossary.

LYCHEE AND PASSION FRUIT SORBET
Quick and Adventurous

173 calories per serving

Prep Time: 10 minutes
Cook Time: 30 minutes

10 lychee nuts,* shelled and pureed = about $^1/_2$ cup
syrup: 2 cups water and one cup sugar
seeds from 2 passion fruits
1 egg white

Shell and puree the lychee. Combine with 2 cups of syrup. Mix the passion fruit seeds with the egg white, and beat until frothy. Combine all the ingredients and place in a sorbet, or ice cream, maker.

Serves 4-6

*Information on this ingredient is included in the Glossary.

GREEN APPLE SORBET WITH STRAWBERRIES AND A BLUEBERRY MERINGUE

Quick and Easy

178 calories per serving

Prep Time: 15 minutes
Cook Time: 30 minutes

$^1/_2$ cup lime or lemon juice
2 cups water
2 apples, quartered, with seeds removed
1 cup simple syrup (see recipe on page 302)
strawberries, small basket
$^1/_2$ cup frozen or fresh blueberries
2 egg whites
$^1/_2$ cup sugar

Note: In order to avoid apples turning brown, combine $^1/_4$ cup lemon or lime juice with 2 cups water, and add apples as soon as they are quartered.

Cut the apples into quarters and remove seeds. Place the apples with the acidulated water on the stove, and poach until they're soft. Lift out the apples with a strainer, and puree with 2 tablespoons of lime or lemon juice. You will have about $^3/_4$ cup of puree. Combine all of the apple puree with one cup simple syrup *plus* 2 tablespoons lemon or lime juice. Place in a sorbet maker. While the sorbet is freezing, beat 2 egg whites lightly in a metal bowl until just frothy. Then add a half cup of sugar and beat well to make the meringue. Puree a half cup blueberries, and combine with the meringue, or serve on top of sorbet. Wash and slice the strawberries.

To serve: Place some of the sorbet on a plate, surround with strawberries, and spoon some meringue artfully around the plate.

Serves 4–6

COFFEE FLAN
Quick and Easy

305 calories per serving

Prep Time: 10 minutes
Cook Time: 45–50 minutes

  $^1/_2$ cup sugar
  4 egg whites
  1 egg
  14 oz. evaporated skim milk
  3 Tbsp. espresso or very strong coffee, cooled
  1 tsp. vanilla
  4 tsp. grated orange rind
  4 tsp. raisins, plumped in $^1/_4$ cup warm water
    (**optional:** use Kahlua!)
  4 tsp. dark chocolate shavings
  2 tsp. ground coffee

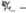

Preheat oven to 350 degrees. Mix together sugar, egg whites, and egg. Whisk in evaporated milk, espresso, and vanilla, and continue whisking until sugar is well dissolved. Pour into 6–8 oz. ramekins. Place ramekins in a baking dish with enough hot water to come midway up their sides.

Bake for 20 minutes. Lower heat to 325 degrees, and gently spoon orange rind and raisins into each ramekin. Continue cooking until a knife comes out clean when inserted into the middle of each ramekin, about 25 minutes more.

Allow to come to room temperature in the water bath. Sprinkle with chocolate and ground coffee, and refrigerate.

Serves 4

A SMOOTHIE
Quick and Easy

183 calories per serving
Prep Time: 5 minutes; Cook Time: 0

> 10 oz. pineapple (1 heaping cup of chunks) about $1/4$ of a
> pineapple or 1 peach, peeled and cut up
> 4 oz. strawberries (1 cup whole), fresh or frozen
> 4 oz. raspberries (1 cup whole), fresh or frozen
> $1/2$ banana
> 1 tsp. vanilla
> $3/4$ cup water
> 1–2 packages artificial sweetener, or
> maple syrup to taste

———————————— ❧ ————————————

Blend all the ingredients except sweetener. Taste for sweetness. Since the fruit varies tremendously in taste, you may not need any added sweetness, or you may want a little more.

———————————— ❧ ————————————

Serves 1 or 2 as a snack or breakfast

VANILLA PEACHES
Quick and Adventurous

69 calories per serving
Prep Time: 10 minutes; Cook Time: 0

4 peaches, sliced	1 cup nonfat yogurt
$1/2$ tsp. vanilla	1 Tbsp. mirin*

———————————— ❧ ————————————

Combine yogurt, vanilla, and mirin. Spoon onto dessert plate, making a lake of the sauce. Arrange peaches on top. Serve.

———————————— ❧ ————————————

Serves 4

*Information on this ingredient is included in the Glossary.

APPLE-PEAR WITH KIWI SAUCE

Quick and Easy

102 calories per serving
Prep Time 10 minutes; Cook Time: 0

5 kiwis	¹/₄ cup maple syrup
2 apple pears	nutmeg

Peel and core the kiwis, and puree. You will have about one cup. Add ¹/₄ cup maple syrup and mix well. Slice and core the apple-pears. Place some sauce on a plate, and top artfully with the apple-pears. Serve with a grind of nutmeg.

Serves 6

PASSION FRUIT COMPOTE

Quick and Adventurous

95 calories per serving
Prep Time: 10 minutes; Cook Time: 0

2 kiwis, peeled and sliced	1 Tbsp. fresh ginger, minced
6 passion fruit*	juice of 1 orange
¹/₄ pineapple, sliced	juice of 1 lime

Scoop out passion fruit and mix well with all other ingredients. Chill and serve.

Serves 4

We know that passion fruit can be expensive, but they are so delicious and low in fat, we think you should give yourself a treat. Besides, this dessert is less expensive than cheesecake!

*Information on this ingredient is included in the Glossary.

Sweets

MANGOES WITH ORANGE SAUCE
Quick and Easy

260 calories per serving
Prep Time: 10 minutes; Cook Time: 10 minutes

juice of 6 oranges
3 mangoes, peeled and sliced
2" fresh ginger, julienned

$^1/_2$ cup maple syrup
2 sprigs mint, chopped

Boil the juice, maple syrup, and ginger for 10 minutes. Cool.
Cover the sliced mangoes with sauce, and sprinkle with mint. A strawberry on top adds a nice touch of color.

Serves 4

A SWEET
Quick and Adventurous

92 calories per serving
Prep Time: 10 minutes; Cook Time: 0

1 mango, skinned and diced
seeds of 4 passion fruits
1 banana, pureed
8 kumquats, diced and seeded

$^1/_3$ cup nonfat plain yogurt
$^1/_4$ tsp. vanilla
1 Tbsp. mint, chopped

Scoop out the insides of the passion fruit, and mix with mango and kumquat. Combine banana puree, yogurt, and vanilla. To serve, spoon banana-yogurt mixture on the bottom of each place. Put a scoop of fruit in the middle, and top with a sprinkling of mint.

Serves 4

BANANA PARFAIT—TWO WAYS
Quick and Easy

#1: 231 calories per serving   **#2** : 266 calories per serving
Prep Time: 10 minutes; Cook Time: Refrigerate

#1:
Per Serving:

1 banana, sliced	$^1/_2$ tsp. vanilla
$^1/_2$ cup nonfat yogurt	1 Tbsp. honey

$^1/_8$ tsp. nutmeg or Chinese Five Spices (Five Spices should be
  available in the spice section of your supermarket)
optional: $^1/_2$–1 pkg. nonsugar sweetener (to your taste)
  mixed in yogurt

Warm one teaspoon honey, and place in a clear glass (a wine glass works well). Swirl until it coats all sides of the glass. Combine the yogurt and vanilla in a bowl. Spoon half of this mixture into the glass. Drizzle a little honey on top, then sprinkle with nutmeg or Five Spices. Gently add slices of half a banana. Repeat the process, adding the last $^1/_4$ cup of yogurt on top with a final sprinkling of spice. Refrigerate at least 30 minutes before serving.

OR

#2:
Per Serving:

1 banana, sliced	1 Tbsp. honey
$^3/_4$ cup nonfat yogurt	2 tsp. Kahlua
1 tsp. ground coffee	

optional: 1 pkg. nonsugar sweetener (to your taste)
  mixed in yogurt

Spoon one teaspoon Kahlua into a glass, and swirl until it lightly coats the sides of the glass. Spoon $^1/_4$ cup yogurt into the bottom of the glass. Add $^1/_4$ teaspoon honey, and sprinkle with a little ground coffee. Place slices from a half banana on top, and spoon on a half teaspoon Kahlua. Repeat the process, adding the last $^1/_4$ cup of yogurt on top with a final drizzle of honey and a sprinkling of ground coffee. Refrigerate or freeze before serving.

Serves one

POACHED DRIED FRUIT
Quick and Adventurous

79 calories per serving

Prep Time: 12 minutes
Cook Time: 30 minutes

> ¹/₄ cup honey
> 4 cups water
> 1 tsp. grated fresh ginger
> 2" cinnamon stick
> 4 whole cloves
> 1 tsp. coriander seeds
> 2 tsp. fennel seeds
> 1 tsp. Five Spice powder
> 2 stalks lemon grass,* chopped (use the bottom 2" above the root)
> zest of 1 lime
> 1 lb. dried mixed fruits, sliced

———————————— ❦ ————————————

Simmer honey and water for three minutes, stirring until dissolved. Add the cinnamon stick, cloves, coriander seeds, fennel seeds, Five Spice powder, and lemon grass, and simmer for 5 minutes. Add the fruit, including the lime zest, and simmer, covered, for 20 minutes or until the fruit is soft. Remove the fruit with a slotted spoon, and strain the liquid. Serve the fruit, and spoon a little of the liquid on top. (May be even better with some chopped mint on top.)

———————————— ❦ ————————————

Serves 6–8

Excellent with a tart sorbet, such as lemon or tea.

*Information on this ingredient is included in the Glossary.

Sauces, Side Dishes, and Other Wonderful Things

Sauces, Side Dishes, and Other Wonderful Things

ROASTED RED PEPPER SAUCE
Quick and Easy

18 calories per serving

Prep Time: 10 minutes
Cook Time: 30 minutes

3 red bell peppers
1 cup homemade nonfat chicken stock (see
    recipe on page 132) or canned nonfat broth
salt and pepper to taste

————————————— ❧ —————————————

Put the red peppers on a cookie sheet under the broiler or in a 450-degree oven, and roast until slightly blackened on all sides. Watch carefully, and turn the peppers as they brown. It will take about 15–20 minutes. Remove blackened skin, seeds, and veins, and discard; puree the flesh until very smooth. Combine it with the chicken broth, and cook over low heat for 10 minutes. Taste for seasoning, and add salt and pepper to taste.

————————————— ❧ —————————————

Serves 4

*This sauce is wonderful with poultry and some fish.
It is beautiful served on the bottom of the plate or spooned
on top.*

LOW-FAT BBQ SAUCE
Adventurous

71 calories per serving

Prep Time: 15 minutes
Cook Time: 45–60 minutes

1½ cups tomatoes (fresh or canned), chopped
1 cup water
3 Tbsp. tomato puree
½ cup apple cider vinegar
⅓ cup Worcestershire sauce
⅓ cup brown sugar
2 tsp. dry mustard
¼ cup molasses
½ onion, chopped
2 cloves garlic, chopped
2 Tbsp. vegetable oil
1 tsp. cumin seed*
½ tsp. salt
1 tsp. Tabasco sauce or more to taste (we use 1 Tbsp. and
a dash of cayenne)

Combine all ingredients, and simmer for 45 minutes to an hour. Add more water if sauce becomes too thick.

Serves 12

This is a traditional but low-fat Southern BBQ sauce. It is perfect for a BBQ sandwich or for use as a dip. Try it as a dip with the Smoked Scallops and Shrimp (see recipe on page 164).

*Information on this ingredient is included in the Glossary.

Sauces, Side Dishes, and Other Wonderful Things

Sauces, Side Dishes, and Other Wonderful Things

CHERMOULA
Quick and Adventurous

27 calories per serving

Prep Time: 10 minutes
Cook Time: 0

1 medium onion, chopped
3 garlic cloves, chopped
2 Tbsp. cilantro,* chopped
2 Tbsp. parsley, chopped
$1/2$ tsp. salt
1 tsp. pepper
1 Tbsp. olive oil
.25 gm (about $1/16$ tsp.) saffron* in 1 Tbsp. hot water
$1/2$ tsp. cumin* powder
1 tsp. paprika

———————————————— ❧ ————————————————

Combine all of the above ingredients and grind to a paste. Makes just less than a cup (about 6 servings)

———————————————— ❧ ————————————————

Makes about one cup

This is one of the infinite variations of the national spice of Morocco. It's sort of used like ketchup, but it's a thousand times better and tastier. It is a flavor enhancer that can be used as a marinade, as a stuffing, and as a condiment. Rub it over some chicken before grilling, or add some after the meat is done.

*Information on this ingredient is included in the Glossary.

RAITA
Quick and Easy

#1: 41 calories per serving
#2: 62 calories per serving

Prep Time: 10 minutes
Cook Time: 0

#1:
2 cups nonfat yogurt
$^1/_2$ cucumber, seeded and thinly sliced
$^1/_4$ red onion, thinly sliced
1 Tbsp. wine vinegar
$^1/_4$ tsp. sugar

Pour the vinegar and sugar over the cucumber and onion. Mix well and allow to sit 5 minutes. Mix with yogurt. Serve in small individual bowls or a larger serving bowl.

OR

#2:
2 cups nonfat yogurt
1 banana, sliced
1 Tbsp. raisins
1 green onion, green part only, sliced
$^1/_2$ tsp. cumin seed*

Combine the banana, raisins, green onion, and cumin seed with yogurt, and serve.

Serves 6–8

Here's an opportunity to be creative and use exactly the ingredients that appeal to you. Raita is an accompaniment to Indian or other spicy foods. The smooth cool yogurt cuts the spice. Some raitas are made of vegetables, others of fruits. Choose your favorites. If you prefer a thinner raita, add a few tablespoons of skim milk.

*Information on this ingredient is included in the Glossary.

Sauces, Side Dishes, and Other Wonderful Things

317

MOCK CHEESE

Easy

31 calories per serving

Prep Time: 2 minutes
Cook Time: overnight

2 cups nonfat yogurt

Strain yogurt through a fine sieve or cheesecloth over into a bowl. Let strain overnight. The liquid strained will be about one cup, and the remaining "cheese," one cup.

Use as a cheese substitute for stuffed chilies, pizza, dips, etc.

Chapter Fifteen

On Your Mark, Get Set, Go!

Look in any bookstore at the health and nutrition section. There you will find hundreds of guides on healthy eating, weight loss, diet, calorie counters, and much more. And in the yellow pages of most cities, you will find a long list of establishments promising weight loss, longer life, better diabetic control, firmer bodies, and good health.

Over the past two decades, the number of health clubs, books, tapes, devices, and videos dealing with health and nutrition has increased exponentially. But despite this surge of interest, the percentage of Americans who are overweight has also increased. We are now the fattest of the First World countries. *Over half* of our population—more than 50 percent—are overweight (as defined by a Body Mass Index over 25). Many overweight Americans are not only fat, but actually obese.

With all of the nutritional help and information available, why are we still getting fatter as a nation? With the advent of the new food pyramid and new labeling laws, why are we continuing to expand our waistlines? And, with the proliferation of theories, diets, and regimens to lose weight and be healthier, why are cancer and heart disease still major health problems?

Certainly the underlying causes are complex, and involve culture, advocacy, advertising, food availability, food types, and other pressures of society and civilization. But it is also obvious that we are doing something wrong in the way we feed ourselves. Hopefully we have helped to explain the problem, and what you can do about it for yourself, your family, and your loved ones.

If you have gotten this far, you are off to a good start and are well on your way to putting into practice what we have said here. When you close this book, you'll find that it wasn't such a hard journey after all. Once you understand the basic principles, the rest is relatively simple.

Having at one time eaten a meat-and-potatoes diet, and having cooked with butter and cream, we understand that the change seems to be a drastic one at first. Yet we assure you that this diet plan is so easy and natural that you will find it difficult to eat a high-fat meal after listening to the instructions of your genes rather than the advertising of fast-food chains.

Follow our clues on how we decide "what to make for dinner tonight." We think that our technique is a fresh, exciting way to plan your menus.

Keep your eye on your heredity, and protect it and yourself by eating well. Reread the guidelines at the end of chapter twelve. Also, take advantage of our society's advanced technology to help keep you healthy and on track.

Good luck, and please let Kathye and me know about your personal evolutionary success.

※ ※ ※ ※ ※ ※

PART III
Appendix

Glossary I

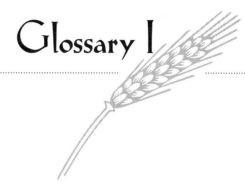

Information on Cooking Terms and Foreign and Exotic Ingredients

AL DENTE: Italian term used in reference to slightly undercooking pasta in order to keep it firm and flavorful. The body of the pasta should be maintained in its original form. When pasta is overcooked, it becomes mushy.

ANAHEIM CHILI: Also known as the California or long green chili, and closely related to the New Mexico chili. Pale to medium bright green, tapered, and measuring about 6 inches long and 2 to 2½ inches in diameter. Medium to thick fleshed; has a green vegetable flavor that is improved by roasting. Originally grown around Anaheim in Southern California at the turn of the 20th century.

ARBORIO RICE: Rice used in making risotto. It is a short- to medium-grained fat rice that absorbs liquid without breaking or becoming mushy. The rice grains hold their shape.

ASAFOETIDA: Obtained from the resinous gum of a plant growing in Afghanistan and Iran, asafoetida has quite an unpleasant smell by itself. Used mainly in Indian cooking and in very small amounts, its main purpose is to prevent flatulence, a useful quality particularly when dried beans and lentils are the main source of protein. Available from Asian and Indian food stores.

BEAN SAUCE: This is a smooth sauce made from fermented soy beans.

BONITO FLAKES: Fish, similar to tuna, which has been dried by salting and airing. The flakes come in light cellophane bags. Pink flakes are preferred to brown flakes. Available in Asian markets.

BULGUR WHEAT: Wheat that has been steamed, dried, and cracked. Available in fine, medium, or coarse grades. Used to make tabbouleh.

CARAWAY SEEDS: Seeds of the *Carum Carvi*, a plant widely distributed throughout Europe and parts of Asia. Used in flavoring.

CARDAMON PODS: Originating in India, cardamon is used as a curry powder blend. Exudes strong, cool, eucalyptus-scented flavor.

CHERVIL: Delicate herb, which should be finely chopped like parsley shortly before adding to dishes. Adds great flavor to chicken, seafood, or vegetable soups. Taste is similar to anise.

CHIPOTLE CHILI: A large, dried, smoked jalapeno; also known as a chili ahumado or a chili meco. Dull tan to coffee brown in color, veined and ridged, measuring about 2 to 4 inches long and about one inch across. Medium thick fleshed, smoky and sweet in flavor with tobacco and chocolate tones, a Brazil nut finish, and a subtle, deep, rounded heat. As much as one-fifth of the Mexican jalapeno crop is processed as chipotles. It is usually available canned.

CILANTRO (CORIANDER): Found in fresh leaves or in dried powder form. Used heavily in Mexican and Indian cooking. Cilantro is the main ingredient in curry powder. Fresh cilantro can be obtained in many supermarkets or in any Mexican or Indian grocer.

COCKLES: Small edible bivalves. Used in place of, or with, mussels, clams, oysters, and crab. Adds great flavor to soups.

COMICE PEARS: French pears that are sweeter, softer, and more fragile than their American counterparts. They are the preferred pear to use in most desserts.

CORIANDER POWDER: The dried and powdered form of Chinese parsley or cilantro.

COUSCOUS: North African dish consisting of coarsely ground wheat, or sometimes semolina pasta. It is prepared by steaming over boiling water.

CRIMINI MUSHROOM: Giant crimini mushrooms are portobello mushrooms. Criminis appear darker in color.

CUMIN: Plant of the carrot family, with crescent-shaped pungent seeds; they look like caraway seeds, but the two are not interchangeable. Essential ingredient in prepared curry.

CUMIN SEED: One of the most commonly used hot spices along with hot peppers. This spice is found in Middle Eastern, Mexican, and Indian foods.

CURRY LEAVES: The flavor from curry leaves is much sought after in South Indian, Sri Lankan, and Malaysian cooking. These compound leaves, which are composed of a number of smaller, shiny leaflets, are used fresh in the tropical countries in which they grow, but outside these regions are mostly available dried. They are added at the start of cooking and give a good flavor. Curry powder is not a substitute for curry leaves.

DAIKON RADISH: Giant Japanese white radish. Grows up to two feet in length. Sliced thin, it is crunchy, sharp, and sweet.

DASHI: Clear Japanese soup made from dried bonito flakes and seaweed. Essential for Japanese cooking and used as stock, soup, or dipping sauce.

DRIED SEAWEED: Made from sea kelp, it is chiefly used as a garnish. Known as Nori in Japan. It is paperlike in consistency and is used for wrapping sushi. Konbu, another variety, is used to make dashi.

ENOKI MUSHROOM: Best used raw in salads or added to soups or other dishes.

ESCOLAR: Large, rough-scaled deep-sea, mackerel-type fish. Lives at depths of 100–400 fathoms (1 fathom = 6 feet). Can be found in the Mediterranean, Atlantic, and Southern seas.

FENUGREEK SEEDS: Small brown seeds that are used in small quantities in curries. They impart a bitter taste, so use only as stated. Available in shops specializing in Indian ingredients.

FISH SAUCE: Thin, salty, brown sauce prepared by packing a variety of fish in barrels and collecting the liquid that runs off. Used primarily in Southeast Asian cooking. Different grades can be found according to country.

GALANGA (also called Laos root): A seasoning with a ginger-pepper taste. Used in East Asian cooking, and sometimes used in place of ginger in Thailand.

HABANERA CHILI: Dark green to orange, orange-red, or red when fully ripe. Lantern shaped, and measuring about 2 inches long and $1^{1}/_{4}$ to $1^{3}/_{4}$ inches in diameter. The habanera (meaning from Havana) is the hottest of any chili grown in Central America or anywhere in the rest of the world. It is estimated to be 30 to 50 times hotter than the jalapeno! Has a distinct flavor with fruity tones. USE WITH CAUTION.

HARISSA: Moroccan hot red pepper sauce.

JALAPENO CHILI: Hot Mexican pepper named for the town of Jalapa in the state of Veracruz, Mexico. When fully ripened and smoked, it becomes a chipotle. Available in most supermarkets with a Mexican produce section.

JAPANESE EGGPLANT: Lavender in color, smaller, and more narrow than its Western counterpart. Its taste is sweeter, it is more tender, and it contains fewer seeds. Ready to be cut and cooked. The eggplant is native to Southeast Asia, not the Mediterranean area as is commonly thought.

JICAMA: Also known as a yam bean. These turnip-shaped tubers are very starchy and are used in salads, Vietnamese spring rolls, and stews.

KONBU: (See "Dried Seaweed).

LEMON GRASS: Used to impart lemony flavor to curries and various Asian dishes. Pull away fibrous outer sheath and discard like corn, and use portion about 5 inches from the root. Slice thin, and chop.

LYCHEE: Tropical Chinese fruit. Crack open lychee nut shells, and peel them away. A pearl-white, plump, sweet fruit is concealed inside.

MIRIN: Japanese rice wine that is sweeter than sake. Substitute dry sherry.

MISO: A paste made from cooked, fermented soy beans. Comes in red, white, brown, or beige. Makes Japanese soup (dashi) thicker. Usually one tablespoon per cup of stock is added. Saltiness will vary.

MOREL MUSHROOM: Also called corncob (Pennsylvania) or sponge mushroom. Somewhat sweet in flavor, it has a yellow hollow head with ribs and combs and a hollow stem.

MUSHROOM SOY SAUCE: Soy sauce flavored with mushrooms.

MUSTARD OIL: Cooking oil widely used in Asia.

NAGE: A sauce that is more liquid and thin, like a soup.

NEW MEXICO CHILI: Also known as the long green chili. Pale to medium green, and red when ripe, tapered, and measuring between 6 to 9 inches long and about $1^1/2$ to 2 inches in diameter. Medium fleshed, it varies considerably in strength from medium to very hot. It has a sweet and earthy flavor and differs from the Anaheim chili in that it is hotter and clearer, with a more cutting chili flavor.

OSTRICH: Swift-running bird that does not fly, which naturally inhabits the plains of Africa and Arabia. It is now raised in the U.S. and is very low in fat (about 18 percent). Tastes like a mild red meat.

OYSTER SAUCE: Prepared by cooking oysters in soy sauce and brine (salt water). Often cornstarch and caramel coloring are added to give it a brown and thick consistency.

PASILLA CHILI: Also known as the chili negro. Literally "little raisin," the pasilla is a dried chilaca chili. There is some confusion over the name of this chili. In California and northern Mexico, the fresh poblano and its dried forms, the anco and mulatto, are referred to as pasillas. It is dark raisin brown, wrinkled, elongated, and tapering. Measuring about 5 to 6 inches long and 1 to 1½ inches across. Thick fleshed; has some berry, grape, and herbaceous tones.

PASSION FRUIT: The edible seeds of some types of passion flower trees. It looks like a brown shriveled egg. Slice it in half and scoop out the delicious tangy seeds.

PORTOBELLO MUSHROOM: Popular large domestic mushroom found in supermarkets. More tasty than the smaller crimini mushrooms. Portobellos are sold when the caps are open and most flavorful. Best for grilling or roasting. The flavor is so intense that it almost tastes like meat.

POUSSIN: A baby chicken, enough for one person. Prepared by grilling to retain juice and flavor.

QUAIL EGGS: The taste is not distinguishable from hens' eggs, but they are about ⅙ the size. Will be kept fresh for two weeks if refrigerated. A staple in Vietnam and Thailand. Found in gourmet stores. They are often used in sushi, or to decorate.

RAMEKIN: Small mold for baking and serving individual portions.

RICE WINE: Also known as sake. Served slightly warmed in tiny cups. Dry white wine is usually the most suitable substitute.

RICE WINE VINEGAR: Staple seasoning throughout most of East Asia (*vinegar* = sour wine in French). Made from rice wine and alcohol, aged, with acetic acid added for aging and bacteria production.

SAFFRON: The world's most expensive spice is obtained by drying the stamens of the saffron crocus. There are only three fragile strands in each flower, and they have to be separated from the petals by hand. It is estimated that 250,000 of the stamens make a kilo of saffron. It only takes a small amount to flavor a dish, and if a small quantity of good saffron is purchased and kept in an airtight container in the freezer, it will keep its flavor for years.

SERRANO CHILI: Dark green to scarlet when ripe. Cylindrical with a tapered, rounded end; measures about 1 to 2 inches long and ½ to ¾ inches in diameter. Thick fleshed; has a clean, biting heat and pleasantly high acidity. Literally "highland" or "mountain," the serrano is one of the hottest chilies commonly available in the United States.

SHIITAKE MUSHROOMS: Large, black, very flavorful Japanese mushrooms with white fissures. Cultivated on the shii tree in Japan. Can be found either fresh or dried.

SHRIMP PASTE: Minced prawns with oil and fish sauce added. It is cut off in slices to be pounded with other seasonings into sauces, dips, and curry pastes. Used as a condiment in Southeast Asian cooking.

TAMARIND: A tropical tree that bears large beans with brittle brown shells. Inside are hard seeds surrounded by a sweet-sour brown pulp that gives a distinctive acid flavor different from lemon juice or vinegar. Tamarind is often sold in dried form with or without the seeds, the shell having been removed. Soak a tablespoonful in a half cup of hot water for a few minutes. Knead and rub with the fingers until the pulp dissolves in the water, then strain out and discard the seeds and fibers. Use the liquid.

It is also possible to purchase jars of ready-to-use concentrate. One or two teaspoons of this tamarind pulp concentrate is equal to 2 rounded tablespoons of dried tamarind when soaked and strained as described above.

TOMATILLO: Mexican gooseberry, sometimes mistakenly called "green tomato"; it delivers a sour tang flavor to dishes. Makes great salsa and other mild Mexican sauces.

TRUFFLE OIL: Made from the rich-flavored fungus that grows underground and has been valued as a delicacy. It is very expensive!

TURKEY CAJUN SAUSAGE: The most distinctive American sausages are Creole or Cajun from Louisiana. Contains minced turkey meat with spices.

TURMERIC: A bright yellow powder used for flavoring and coloring curries and other Indian and Southeast Asian dishes. Turmeric is related to the ginger family.

UNI: A sea urchin. Usually eaten raw, it has a delicious, strong flavor. Used as a flavor enhancer.

WASABI: Pungent, green horseradish used in Japanese cooking. Available dried and powdered in tins. Reconstituted, like dry mustard, by adding cold water. Often served with ginger when eating sushi or sashimi.

WOOD EAR MUSHROOM: Sold dried in Asian grocery stores. The mushroom bloats up when soaked in warm water. Best served as a "crunchy" accompaniment to most dishes such as stir-fry meals.

YAMAGOBO: Edible pickled burdock roots. Looks like a carrot on a diet. Very interesting flavor.

YAM NOODLES: Noodles made from Japanese yams.

❇ ❇ ❇ ❇ ❇ ❇

Glossary II

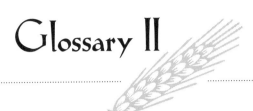

Mail-Order Resources for Foreign and Hard-to-Find Foods

FRESH AND FROZEN ORIENTAL FOODS
Anzen Oriental Foods and Imports
736 N.E. MLK Jr. Boulevard
Portland, OR 97232
(503) 233-5111
FAX (503) 233-7208

ALL KINDS OF SMOKED FISH AND CAVIAR
Barney Greengrass,
  the Sturgeon King
541 Amsterdam Avenue
New York, NY 10024
(212) 724-4707

CHILIES, TAMALES, AND OTHER SOUTHWESTERN FOODS
Bueno Foods
2001 Fourth Street, S.W.
Albuquerque, NM 87102
(505) 243-2722

CHILIES AND CHILI PRODUCTS
The Chile Shop
109 E. Water Street
Santa Fe, NM 87501
(505) 983-6080

HARD-TO-FIND INGREDIENTS FROM ALL OVER THE WORLD
The CMC Company
P.O. Box Drawer B
Avalon, NJ 08202
(800) CMC-2780
FAX (609) 861-0043

GAME BIRDS, DUCK, GAME
D'Artagnan, Inc.
399-419 St. Paul Avenue
Jersey City, NJ 07306
(800) DARTAGN

**UNUSUAL FRUITS
AND VEGETABLES**
Frieda's Inc.
P.O. Box 58488
Los Angeles, CA 90058
(800) 241-1771

**SEEDS, HERBS,
AND PLANTS**
Le Jardin du Gourmet
P.O. Box 75
St. Johnsbury Center, VT 05863
(802) 748-1446

**CHILIES AND OTHER SOUTH-
WESTERN PRODUCTS**
Los Chileros De Nuevo Mexico
P.O. Box 6215
Santa Fe, NM 87502
(505) 471-6967

**ALL KINDS OF RICE
PRODUCTS**
Lundberg Family Farms
5370 Church Street
P.O. Box 369
Richvale, CA 95974-0369
(916) 882-4551

**EUROPEAN FOODS, STOCKS,
AND DRIED MUSHROOMS**
Midwest Imports
1121 South Clinton
Chicago, IL 60607
(312) 939-8400

**GREAT VARIETY OF ASIAN
FOODS AND CONDIMENTS**
Oriental Food Market and
  Cooking School, Inc.
Chu-Yen and Pansy Like
2801 W. Howard Street
Chicago, IL 60645
(312) 274-2826

ASIAN GROCERIES
The Oriental Pantry
423 Great Road
Acton, MA 01720
(800) 828-0368
(508) 264-4576

**MIDDLE EASTERN,
MOROCCAN, AND INDIAN
FOOD PRODUCTS**
Sahadi
187-189 Atlantic Avenue
Brooklyn, NY 11201
(718) 624-4550

**ALL KINDS OF HERBS
AND SPICES**
San Francisco Herb Co.
250 14th Street
San Francisco, CA 94103
(800) 227-4530 or (415) 861-7174

**WIDE VARIETY OF INDIAN AND
ASIAN PRODUCTS**
Spice Merchant
P.O. Box 524
Jackson Hole, WY 83001
(800) 551-5999

ASIAN PRODUCTS
Uwajimaya
519 Sixth Avenue S.
Seattle, WA 98104
(206) 624-6248

❈ ❈ ❈ ❈ ❈

Citations

(This is a partial list of an enormous bibliography. If you wish the full list of citations, please contact the authors through Hay House.)

BREAST

Howe, G. R. "Dietary fat and breast cancer risks. An epidemiologic perspective." *Cancer* **74** (3 Suppl.) (1994): 1078-1084.

van den Brandt, P. A. et al. " A prospective cohort study on dietary fat and the risk of postmenopausal breast cancer," *Cancer Res.* **53** (1993): 75-82.

Wynder, E. L., D. P. Rose and L. A. Cohen. "Diet and Breast Cancer in Causation and Therapy," *Cancer* **58** (1986): 1804-1813.

INSULIN

Pyorala, K. "Hyperinsulinaemia as predictor of atherosclerotic vascular disease: epidemiological evidence," *Diabetes Metab.* **17** France: (1991): 87-92.

Sowers, J. R. et al. "Hyperinsulinemia, insulin resistance, and hyperglycemia: contributing factors in the pathogenesis of hypertension and atherosclerosis," *American Journal of Hypertension* **6** (1993): 260S—270S.

UPPER AIRWAY

La Vecchia, C. et al. "Dietary indicators of oral and pharyngeal cancer," *International Journal of Epidemiology* **20** (1991): 39-44.

LUNG

Alavanja, M. C. et al. "Saturated fat intake and lung cancer risk among non-smoking women in Missouri," *Journal of the National Cancer Institute* **85** (1993): 1906-1916.

Marchand, L. L. et al. "Intake of Specific Carotenoids and Lung Cancer Risk," *Cancer Epidemiology, Biomarkers & Prevention* **2** (1993): 183-187.

PROSTATE

Pienta, K. J. and P. S. Esper. "Is Dietary Fat a Risk Factor for Prostate Cancer?" *Journal of the National Cancer Institute* **85** (1993): 2538-1540.

Whittenmore, A. S. et al. "Prostate Cancer in Relation to Diet, Physical Activity, and Body Size in Blacks, Whites, and Asians in the United States and Canada," *Journal of the National Cancer Institute* **87** (1995):652-661.

COLON

Giovannucci, E. et al. "Intake of fat, meat, and fiber in relation to risk of colon cancer in men," *Cancer Res.* **54** (1994): 2390-2397.

Henderson, M. M. "International differences in diet and cancer incidence," *Monogr. Natl. Cancer Inst.* (1992): 59-63.

Thun, M. J., M. M. Namboodiri and C. W. Heath, Jr. "Aspirin Use and Reduced Risk of Fatal Colon Cancer" *The New England Journal of Medicine* **325** (1991): 1593-1596.

GASTRIC

Graham, S. et al. "Diet in the epidemiology of gastric cancer," *Nutr. Cancer* **13** (1990): 19-34.

Ramon, J. M. et al. "Dietary Factors and Gastric Cancer Risk," *Cancer* **71** (1993): 1731-1735.

ESOPHAGUS

Funkhouser, E. M. and G. B. Sharp. "Aspirin and Reduced Risk of Esophageal Carcinoma," *Cancer* **76** (1995): 1116-1119.

Ghadirian, P., J. M. Ekoe and J. P. Thouez. "Food habits and esophageal cancer: an overview," *Cancer Detect Prev.* **16** (1992): 163-168.

OVARY

Engle, A., J. E. Muscat and R. E. Harris. "Nutritional risk factors and ovarian cancer," *Nutr. Cancer* **15** (1991): 239-247.

Risch, H. A. et al. "Dietary Fat Intake and Risk of Epithelial Ovarian Cancer," *Journal of the National Cancer Institute* **86** (1994): 1409-1415.

INFANTS AND CHILDREN

Hardy, S. C. and R. E. Kleinman. "Fat and cholesterol in the diet of infants and young children: implications for growth, development, and long-term health," *J. Pediatr.* **125** (5 Pt. 2) (1994): S69-77.

Haust, M. D. "The genesis of atherosclerosis in pediatric age-group," *Pediatr. Pathol.* **10** (1990): 253-271.

Rocchini, A. P. "Fetal and pediatric origins of adult cardiovascular disease," *Curr. Opin. Pediatr.* **6** (1994): 591-595.

HUNTER-GATHERER

Eaton, S. B., M. Shostak and M. Konner. *The Paleolithic Prescription.* New York: Harper & Row, 1988.

Mancilha-Carvalho, J. J. and D. E. Crews. "Lipid profiles of Yanomamo Indians of Brazil," *Prev. Med.* 19 (1990): 66-75.

Tanaka, J., D.W. Hughes. *The SAN Hunter-Gatherers of the Kalahari.* Tokyo: University of Tokyo Press, 1980.

MORMONS AND ADVENTISTS

Lyon, J. L., K. Gardner and R. E. Gress. "Cancer incidence among Mormons and non-Mormons in Utah (United States) 1971-1985," *Cancer Causes Control* **5** England: (1994): 149-156.

Mills, P. K. et al. "Cancer incidence among California Seventh-Day Adventists, 1976-1982," *Am. J. Clin. Nutr.* **59** (5 Suppl) (1994): 1136S-1142S.

Mills, P. K. et al. "Cohort study of diet, lifestyle, and prostate cancer in Adventist men," *Cancer* **64** (1989): 598-604.

ANTIOXIDANTS AND CANCER

Byers, T. and N. Guerrero. "Epidemiologic evidence for vitamin C and vitamin E in cancer prevention," *Am. J. Clin. Nutr.* **62** (6 Suppl) 1385S-1392S.

Hennekens, C. H. "Antioxidant vitamins and cancer," *Am. J. Med.* **97** (3A) (1994): 2S-4S, 22S-28S.

VITAMIN C

Block, G. "Vitamin C and cancer prevention: the epidemiologic evidence," *Am. J. Clin. Nutr.* **53** (1 Suppl) (1991): 270S-282S.

Dorgan, J. F. and A. Schatzkin. "Antioxidant micronutrients in cancer prevention," *Hematol. Oncol. Clin.* **5** England: (1991): 43-68.

ESKIMOS

Newman, W. P. et al. "Atherosclerosis in Alaska Natives and non-natives," *Lancet* **341** England: (1993): 1056-1057.

VITAMIN E

Das, S. "Vitamin E. in the genesis and prevention of cancer. A review," *Acta. Oncol.* **33** Norway: (1994): 615-619.

DIET-PREVENTION

Schapira, D. V. "Nutrition and cancer prevention," *Prim. Care* 19 (1992): 481-491. Carroll, K. K. "Dietary fats and cancer," *Am. J. Clin. Nutr.* **53** (4 Suppl) (1991): 1064S-1067S.

Weinhouse, Sidney. "The Role of Diet and Nutrition in Cancer," *Cancer* **58** (1986): 1791-1794.

EGGS

Cobb, M. M. and H. Teitlebaum. "Determinants of plasma cholesterol responsiveness to diet," *Br. J. Nutr.* **71** England: (1994): 271-282.

Cox, C. et al. "Individual variation in plasma cholesterol response to dietary saturated fat," *B. M. J.* **311**, England: (1995): 1260-1264.

Knuiman, J. T. et al. "Total cholesterol and high density lipoprotein cholesterol levels in populations differing in fat and carbohydrate intake," *Arteriosclerosis* **7** (1987): 612-619.

INFANT NUTRITION

Finberg, L. "Modified fat diets: do they apply to infancy?" *J. Pediatr.* **117** (1990) S132-S133.

Lapinleimu, H. et al. "Prospective randomized trial in 1062 infants of diet low in saturated fat and cholesterol," *Lancet* **345** England (1995): 471-476.

BREAST MILK

Farquharson, J., et al. "Infant cerebral cortex phospholipid fatty-acid composition and diet," *Lancet* **340** England: (1992): 810-813.

Finley, D.A., et al. "Breast milk composition: fat content and fatty acid composition in vegetarians and non-vegetarians," *Am. J. Clin. Nutr.* **41** (1985): 787-800.

Garza, C., et al. "Special properties of human milk," *Clin. Perinatol.* **14** (1987): 11-32.

Jensen, R.G., A.M. Ferris, and C.J. Lammi-Keefe. "Lipids in human milk and infant formulas," *Annu. Rev. Nutr.* **12** (1992): 417-441.

DIETARY CHOLESTEROL

Clarkson, T. B. et al. "Mechanisms of atherogenesis," *Circulation* **76** (1987): 120-128.

Stone, N. J. "Diet, Lipids, and coronary heart disease," *Endocrinol. Metab. Clin. North Am.* **19** (1990): 321- 344.

ASPIRIN AND CANCER

Giovannucci, E, et. al. "Aspirin and the risk of colorectal cancer in women," *N. Engl. J. Med.* **333** (1995): 609-614.

Paganini-Hill, A. "Aspirin and colorectal cancer: the Leisure World cohort revisited," *Prev. Med.* **24** (1995): 113-115.

❆ ❆ ❆ ❆ ❆ ❆

Index

Pages with photos are in bold.

main dishes—fish, shellfish
  BBQ swordfish, 94, 262
  Cajun catfish with marinade, 258
  Cajun dirty rice with shrimp, 249
  Chilean sea bass with papaya coulis and jicama salsa, 268
  crab with black bean sauce, 250
  crab sandwiches, open-faced, 246
  curried fish, 257
  fillet of sole with lime marinade, 255
  grilled fish with mussel shiitake broth, 264
  grilled salmon with Japanese spices, 269
  grilled shrimp with ginger tamarind relish, 251
  grilled swordfish with tomato sauce, 64, 263
  halibut pot au feu, 266-267
  Moroccan shrimp and scallops in chermoula nage, 248
  paella, 252-253
  roasted red snapper with tomatillo salsa, 260
  Shanghai catfish, 259
  spicy mussels, 247
  steamed fish, 254
  Thai-style red snapper, 261
  whitefish with orange tomato sauce, 265
mango
  with orange sauce, 310
  and pumpkin adobo with ostrich oyster steak, 292-293
  sauce with grilled veal cutlet, 299
  and strawberry sorbet, **156**, 302
  in a sweet, 310
marinade
  Asian style, 300
  BBQ, 262
  Cajun, 258
  chermoula, 316
  chermoula nage, 248
  for chicken Bali-H'ai, 278
  chipotle nage, **151**, 294
  lime, 255
  for quail, 284, 285
  for roasted turkey or chicken, 272
  smoked, 164
meat
  "bad" vs. "good," 39-45
    high fat/high saturation, 40-41
    low fat/low saturation, 42-44
  breaded and fat, 46
  domesticated red
    elimination of, 22, 40
    and fat content, 9, 38
    feeding and raising practices, 37-38
    Japanese Kobe beef, 38
  low in fat, 5-6

reducing fat content, 45-46
See also specific types; wild game
menus
from around the world, 124-127
sample seven-day, 88-94
meringue, blueberry, **156**, 306
metabolic function, 2, 5, 11
of cholesterol and carrier fats, 18-19
insulin and sugar, 52-53
milk. See dairy products
miso with broiled clams and sake, 165
Mormons, diet of, 7
mushrooms
enoki in spicy seafood soup, 196
with pearl pasta, 237
portobello and barley soup, 90, **145**, 186
portobello, grilled with sauce, 225
shiitake broth with grilled fish, 264
shiitake open-faced sndwiches, 177
shiitake and wood ear in ravioli, 178-179
wild, on polenta toast, 226-227
mussels
in paella, 252-253
spicy, 247

N

nage. See marinade
Noble Carrot Principle, 122-123

O

oils, 23-24, 25
orange
grapefruit, and fennel salad, 93, **148**, 202
tomato sauce, 265
ostrich, 44
Bolognese, 291
meatloaf with corn adobo, 288-289
meatloaf, traditional, 290
oyster steak with pumpkin/mango adobo, 292-293
roasted in chipotle marinade over creamy polenta, **151**, 294
ovarian cancer, 109
oysters
Julia with dashi, 166
seafood packs, 167

P

pan roasting and fat reduction, 45
papaya

About the Authors

Ronald Citron, M.D., makes no bones about it—he's a great cook. "I learned at the School of Burnt Butter," says the successful oncologist/hematologist. Growing up in New York City, the kitchen was always the warmest room in the house, so he spent most of his free time there. After attending NYU Medical School, he spent two years in Switzerland at the prestigious Institute for Immunology in Basel, doing basic research on cell growth and metabolism. France was, of course, right across the border, and his love of French cooking and wines grew each time he visited there.

After years of successful practice as a Board-certified oncologist and internist, Dr. Citron realized he had seen too many people die needlessly of cancer and heart disease. Their life styles, and especially their eating habits, were killing them. He decided that he could do more good *preventing* cancer and heart disease rather than trying to help a patient when it was already too late.

After creating ***THE CLINICAL COMPUTER: Your Personal Health Manager***, a risk-management program for cancer and heart disease, he realized that the little cookbook included with the program was as popular as the program itself. He sold the computer program (it's now included in a large CD-ROM health program) in order to be able to concentrate on creating the Evolutionary Diet and recipes that are healthy and delicious.

❊ ❊ ❊

The fine cooking of her Southern mother and grandmother sparked a lifelong interest in cuisine for **Kathye J. Citron.** After studying cooking in the U.S. and France, she hosted a daily radio show in Northern California called "What's Cooking." She taught the cooking of several cuisines in Southern California and was owner and executive chef of the successful Los Angeles catering firm "Great Beginnings...Happy Endings."

In the 1980s, Kathye sold her business and became the Executive Director of a Los Angeles nonprofit corporation and then a business consultant.

Her partnership with Dr. Citron and her return to the food industry began in 1990. Since then, Kathye's interest in cuisine has turned to delicious, healthy cooking. Together, the Citrons have traveled extensively, testing the best of French, Italian, Indian, and other world cuisines. Currently, Kathye applies her craft to extracting the true flavors of these cuisines without the use of high-fat ingredients.

❊ ❊ ❊

Both Citrons are members of the James Beard Foundation (Food and Wine Professionals category), the International Wine and Food Society, and the National Restaurant Association.

❊ ❊ ❊

If you would like to contact Ron and Kathye Citron, please write to them in care of Hay House.

❊ ❊ ❊ ❊ ❊ ❊

2409